Practical Laparoscopy

Practical Laparoscopy

G. Berci MD, FACS
Associate Director of Surgery
Cedars–Sinai Medical Center and
Clinical Professor of Surgery
UCLA School of Medicine
Los Angeles, California

A. Cuschieri MD, ChM, FRCS(Ed.), FRCS(Eng.)
Professor and Head of Department of Surgery
Ninewells Hospital and Medical School
University of Dundee;
Consultant Surgeon to the Tayside Health Board
Dundee, Scotland

With contributions on gynaecological laparoscopy by
Geoffrey Chamberlain MD, FRCS, FRCOG
Professor of Obstetrics and Gynaecology
St George's Hospital Medical School
London

and on documentation for laparoscopy by
Margaret Paz-Partlow MA, MFA
Clinical Project Associate, Division of Surgical Endoscopy
Department of Surgery
Cedars–Sinai Medical Center
Los Angeles, California

Baillière Tindall   London Philadelphia Toronto
Mexico City Rio de Janeiro Sydney Tokyo Hong Kong

Baillière Tindall W.B. Saunders	1 St Anne's Road Eastbourne, East Sussex BN21 3UN, England
	West Washington Square Philadelphia, PA 19105, USA
	1 Goldthorne Avenue Toronto, Ontario M8Z 5T9, Canada
	Apartado 26370—Cedro 512 Mexico 4, DF Mexico
	Rua Evaristo da Veiga 55,20° andar Rio de Janeiro—RJ, Brazil
	ABP Australia Ltd, 44–50 Waterloo Road North Ryde, NSW 2113, Australia
	Ichibancho Central Building, 22–1 Ichibancho Chiyoda-ku, Tokyo 102, Japan
	10/fl, Inter-Continental Plaza, 94 Granville Road Tsim Sha Tsui East, Kowloon, Hong Kong

First published 1986

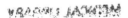

Typeset by Scribe Design, Gillingham, Kent
Printed and bound in Great Britain by Mackays of Chatham

British Library Cataloguing in Publication Data

Berci, G.
    Practical laparoscopy.
    1. Abdomen—Diseases—Diagnosis
    2. Laparoscopy
    I. Title   II. Cuschieri, A.   III. Chamberlain,
    Geoffrey, *1930*–   IV. Paz-Partlow, Margaret
    617'.5507545   RC944

ISBN 0 7020 1132 0

Contents

Colour plates follow p. 104

Introduction

It is now more than 70 years since Kelling and Jacobeus published their experience with laparoscopy in man. Since then this extremely useful clinical procedure has been fully exploited by gynaecologists in both the diagnosis and the management of their patients and it was crucial to the development of in-vitro fertilization. Although laparoscopy has been received enthusiastically by some hepatologists over the past four decades, its use in gastroenterology, general surgery and medicine has been fragmented and ill-defined. Recently, however, laparoscopy has gained favour, as a result of technological advances in optics, light transmission and television display and the introduction of miniature ultrasonic probes and laparoscopic laser techniques.

The procedure is certainly cost-effective, has a high overall diagnostic yield, and has an excellent safety record. Laparoscopy allows direct visualization of the abdominal organs and the peritoneal lining. It permits safe target biopsy or cytology of diseased organs. With experience, the interpretation of laparoscopic findings is easy. Its practical value in the assessment of the degree of advancement of disease is best exemplified by the reduction in the number of unnecessary laparotomies for non-resectable malignant disease which follows the use of laparoscopy in the management of these unfortunate patients. There are few diagnostic modalities which yield as much information on the state of the liver as laparoscopy, and this is well recognized by hepatologists. To the general surgeon and gastroenterologist laparoscopy often provides the answer to diagnostic dilemmas, for example in pyrexia of unknown origin, unexplained abdominal pain or weight loss, ascites of unknown origin and undiagnosed abdominal mass. Often the procedure is used to verify information obtained by more expensive diagnostic techniques such as CT and isotope scanning.

As with all invasive procedures, however, a good training programme in the use of laparoscopy is essential if one is to obtain an overall benefit in terms of patient care. Although there are well established training programmes for flexible fibre-optic endoscopy, only the specialty of obstetrics and gynaecology incorporates laparoscopy as an essential component of the curriculum. The increasing use of laparoscopy in gastroenterology and surgery must be accompanied by an adequate training and audit programme.

This book has been written because there is no introductory manual which emphasizes the technique and practical usage of laparoscopy despite several excellent currently available and well known colour atlases. Our aim has been to cover the practical details of instrumentation and the procedural steps of laparoscopy and its ancillary techniques. As such the book is intended for the beginner and is not a comprehensive reference manual on the subject. Practical steps in the performance of laparoscopy are thus covered in detail, whereas the descriptions of the normal anatomy and the commonly encountered disorders are only outlined. This book is intended to complement clinical training in laparoscopy and is no substitute for supervised clinical experience with the procedure.

We are grateful to our publishers for their courtesy and help during the production of this book and in particular to Mr Seán Duggan for his helpful advice in its preparation. We would also like to thank our two contributors, Professor G. Chamberlain and Mrs M. Paz-Partlow, for their excellent chapters, which helped to complete this monograph and cover areas of special expertise. Finally we are indebted to our secretaries Mrs J. Mackenzie and Mrs A. Wasser for their assistance.

G. Berci, Los Angeles
A. Cuschieri, Dundee

Historical notes

The first reported attempt to inspect the abdominal cavity through a stab incision by introducing a cystoscope was reported by Kelling in 1901 in the dog. Experience in man was published by the same author in 1923.[1] Jacobeus gave an account of his first satisfactory examination of the abdomen in 1910 in patients with ascites. One year later he had performed 115 cases, with one serious complication (bleeding) requiring exploration.[2]

Korbsch extended the indication for its use to include other intra-abdominal disorders in 1922.[3] Steiner reported his first successful 'abdominoscopy' in 1924.[4] In the same year, Zollikofer in Switzerland also claimed success with this examination.[5] In 1933 Fervers reviewed his experience with 50 patients and recommended changing from room air to oxygen or CO_2 as an insufflating agent,[6] while in 1938 Veress invented his spring-loaded needle, which became the instrument of choice to create a pneumoperitoneum.[7]

The real impetus for modern laparoscopy emanated from the work of the hepatologist Kalk, who introduced purpose-designed instruments and in 1929 was the first to advocate the dual-trocar technique.[8] This opened the way for diagnostic and therapeutic laparoscopy. He accumulated an experience of over 2000 cases, with impressive results, and published a monograph on this subject in 1951.[9]

In the United States Ruddock drew attention to this important diagnostic aid and reported on 500 cases in the thirties[10,11] Zoeckler enthusiastically advocated this procedure in 1958, with a series of 1000 cases with a mortality of 0.03%.[12] It took some time until laparoscopy became accepted and routinely employed by gastroenterologists in Europe. During the sixties the impetus was maintained by gynaecologists such as Palmer, Frangenheim, Semm and Steptoe, who contributed to a wider acceptance of this procedure in patients with pelvic pathology.

Beck, Boyce, Jensen, Lindner,[13] Lightdale, Reynolds, Smith, Villardel, Wannagat and Hemmling established the value and safety of laparoscopy in the management of patients with gastroenterological and hepatic disorders. Surgeons have been reluctant to use this procedure until relatively recently. In the USA Berci and Gaisford have been instrumental in demonstrating the therapeutic potential of laparoscopy in general surgical practice and in patients with hepato-biliary disorders. Francis Stock was the first surgeon in the UK to use laparoscopy routinely in general surgical practice and introduced A. Cuschieri to the technique in 1964.

REFERENCES

1 Kelling, G. (1923) Zur Colioskopie. *Arch. klin. Chir. 126:* 226–229
2 Jacobeus, H.C. (1911) Kurze Übersicht über meine Erfahrungen mit der Laparoskopie. *Münch. med. Wschr. 58:* 2017–2019
3 Korbsch, R. (1922) Technik und Grenzen der Laparoskopie. *Münch. med. Wschr. 69:* 426–427
4 Steiner, O.P. (1924) Abdominoskopie. *Schweiz. med. Wschr. 54:* 84–87
5 Zollikofer, R. (1924) Zur Laparoskopie. *Schweiz. med. Wschr. 54:* 264–265
6 Fervers, C. (1933) Die Laparoskopie mit dem Zystoskope. *Medsche Klin. 29:* 1042–1045
7 Veress, J. (1938) Neues Instrument zur Ausführung von Brust oder Bauchpunktionen. *Dt. med. Wschr. 41:* 1480–1481
8 Kalk, H. (1929) Erfahrungen mit der Laparoskopie. *Z. klin. Med. 111:* 303–348
9 Kalk, H. & Bruhl, W. (1951) *Leitfaden der Laparoskopie.* Stuttgart: Thieme.
10 Ruddock, J.C. (1937) Peritoneoscopy. *Surgery Gynec. Obstet. 65:* 523–539
11 Ruddock, J.C. (1934) Peritoneoscopy. *West. J. Surg. Obstet. Gynec. 42:* 392–394
12 Zoeckler, S.J. (1958) Peritoneoscopy. A revaluation. *Gastroenterology 34:* 969–980
13 Lindner, H. (1965) Fortschritte der Photolaparoskopie. *Medsche Welt. 27:* 1513–1519

1
Instrumentation

GENERAL INFORMATION

Before purchasing equipment, which is available from a number of manufacturers, one should become acquainted with a few important principles of image transmission as well as essential features relating to the use of certain accessories.

The telescope

Nitze, a general practitioner, invented the telescope in 1875 and produced the first cystoscope for the examination of the urinary bladder. Small lenses with air interspaces acted as a relay, transmitting the image from the interior of the organ to the eye of the examiner. For illumination (before Edison's invention of the electric light bulb) he employed a glowing platinum wire to light up the interior, but later replaced this cumbersome system with a miniature low-voltage electric bulb.

The Nitze system remained essentially unchanged for several decades. The individual optical elements were improved but the substantial light absorption of the system (90–95%) and its narrow viewing angle, poor colour reproduction and low resolution resulted in a relatively dim, unsatisfactory image. The size of the telescope was limited by the available technology, which precluded the production of smaller lenses. Permanent film records, which require much more light, were difficult, if not impossible, to obtain. Despite the obvious optical shortcomings, endoscopy made its debut in the field of urology and was then extended to broncho-oesophagoscopy and laparoscopy.

A milestone was the invention of the Hopkins rod-lens (Figure 1.1). Instead of transmitting light through a lens–air interspace–lens system, the light beam was guided through a series of glass rods on the ends of which small lenses were cemented. The Hopkins rod-lens system has the following advantages:

1 Light transmission is increased thanks to decreased absorption. Clinically, this results in a brighter image, providing easier perception.

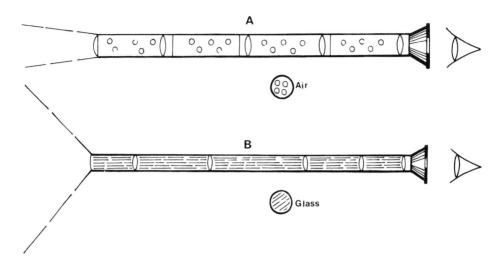

Fig. 1.1 Schematic diagram of telescope. A: standard lens system. Small optical elements are placed at intervals along the cylinder. B: The Hopkins rod lenses. Glass rods replace the previous air intervals.

2   The viewing angle is increased and a larger object image is seen within a single viewing field, resulting in faster orientation.

3   The rod-lens system, with its increased light transmission, allows the production of smaller telescopes, and this enables new areas such as pediatrics or emergency laparoscopy, where very small instruments are required, to be explored. These objectives could not have been achieved using standard lenses.

4   The attributes of the Hopkins system, e.g. the larger viewing angle with simultaneous maximum object enlargement, higher resolution, flat field and excellent colour reproduction allowed photographic documentation and more recently, video recording of intra-abdominal pathology observed by laparoscopy.

The light source

The electric bulb at the distal end of a telescope is nowadays of historical interest. With the advent of flexible fibre-optic transmission, light sources can be placed at a remote location. For routine examination a 150W halogen bulb with a mirror is sufficient (Figure 1.2). High-intensity units are needed for photolaparoscopy, video recording and when a teaching attachment is used. Quartz, mercury or xenon light units are available.

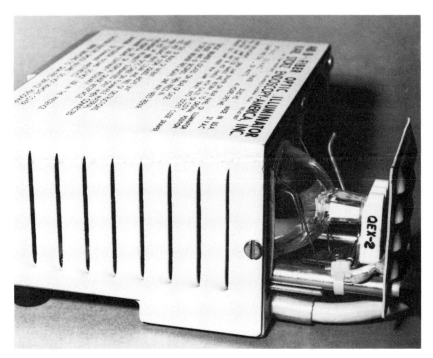

Fig. 1.2 A 150 W halogen bulb with a mirror provides enough illumination for routine examination. The bulb can be replaced with ease.

The fibre-optic light cable

An incoherent fibre-optic cable is plugged in at one end of the light source while the other end is connected to the fibres surrounding the telescope. In this way the light energy is transmitted into the body cavity.

The term 'cold light' is a misnomer because a significant amount of heat is produced at the working end of the fibre-optic cable. This can be tested in a simple manner. Adjust your examining light unit for maximum output and direct the light beam onto your wrist. In a few seconds you will feel pain. Burn injuries do not occur during laparoscopy because the fibres in the instrument surrounding the telescope are fewer in number. Light intensity is further lost during conduction and the heat is distributed over a larger surface (Figure 1.3). In those instruments where more light fibres are packed, e.g., the photolaparoscope, the examiner should be careful to avoid touching the surface of organs with the telescope. This applies only during the use of *continuous* high-intensity light units with maximum output, as during television monitoring or cinematography.

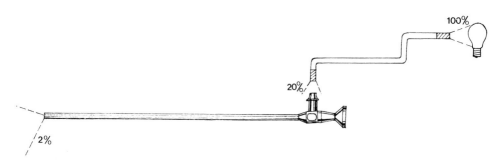

Fig. 1.3 The remotely placed light source provides adequate illumination. An interposed six-foot (1.8 m) flexible fibre bundle absorbs approximately 80% of the light energy. Further absorption occurs in the light fibres which surround the telescope. In general the final light output at the tip of the working end of the scope is not more than 2%.

The fibre-optic cable, though convenient, is a very inefficient transmitter because it absorbs approximately 80% of the input (Figure 1.3). The blue part of the colour spectrum is not well transmitted and the red part of the light spectrum is compressed. This is one of the reasons why some organs look brown or yellowish. Despite these shortcomings it is distinctly superior to the outdated distal electric bulb system.

The fluid cable is a recent innovation. It consists of plastic tubes filled with a special fluid. Both ends of the tubes are sealed with quartz glass plugs. It is less flexible than the glass fibre bundle but light absorption is less and the entire colour spectrum is transmitted, providing excellent natural colour display. Clearly, for the purpose of documentation the fluid bundle is better than the glass fibre bundle.

Accessories

One should ensure that the instruments are of the right quality. Individual items should be properly finished, jaw movements smooth, valves and stopcocks easy to remove, and so on. Containers should be supplied with the instruments.

Before purchasing laparoscopic sets be sure that you know what you are buying and what the prerequisite parameters for optimum performance are. The after-sales service provided is an important practical consideration. Service should be immediately available and details such as cost, replacement instruments etc. clarified before the order is signed.

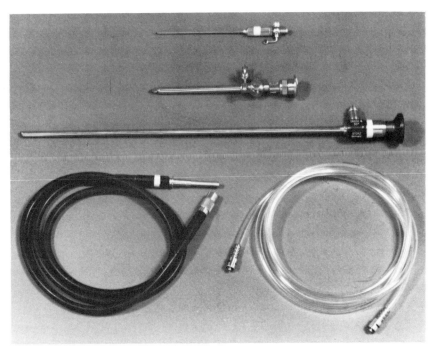

Fig. 1.4   The basic set. From top to bottom: (i) Veress pneumoperitoneum needle. (ii) 7 mm examining cannula with stylet and stopcock; (iii) telescope with the Hopkins rod-lens system and 30° forward-oblique direction of view (we prefer the forward-oblique viewing telescope to the 0° or straight forward viewing one since the upper abdomen and liver especially and other organs generally can be more easily and thoroughly visualized); (iv) the fibre-optic cable and the connecting tube to the insufflator.

THE BASIC SET (Figure 1.4)

The pneumoperitoneum needle

Any type of needle can be used but the Veress needle has distinct advantages. The pneumoperitoneum needle developed by Veress in 1933 has an outer sheath or needle of 2 mm diameter, a spring-loaded hollow *blunt* stylet with a side hole and a Luer female attachment with a stopcock (Figure 1.5). When penetrating through solid tissue, e.g., the abdominal wall, the stylet will be pushed back inside the sheath of the needle (Figure 1.6A,B). As soon as the sharp tip enters the peritoneal cavity the spring pushes out the blunt stylet with an audible click (Figure 1.6C). With further movements of this needle the blunt tip protruding through the needle shaft avoids inadvertent

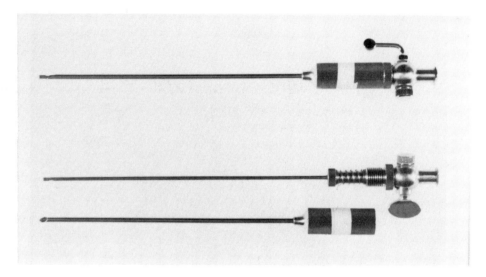

Fig. 1.5   Top: the Veress pneumoperitoneum needle assembled. Bottom: the unassembled needle and the spring-loaded blunt stylet.

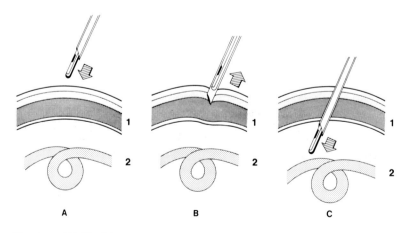

Fig. 1.6   (A) The blunt stylet is protruding and is advanced through a stab incision. 1 = layers of abdominal wall; 2 = intestine. (B) During penetration of the various layers the blunt stylet is pushed back into the needle. (C) As soon as the needle enters a cavity the blunt stylet is pushed forward by the spring action; the blunt end prevents injury.

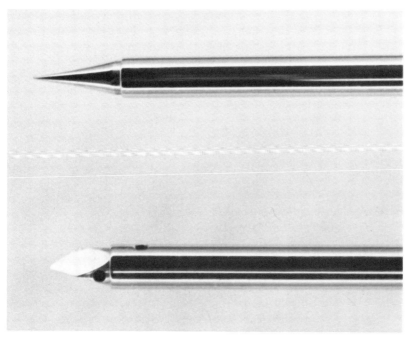

Fig. 1.7a Top: Cone-shaped trocar tip; bottom: pyramid-shaped trocar tip.

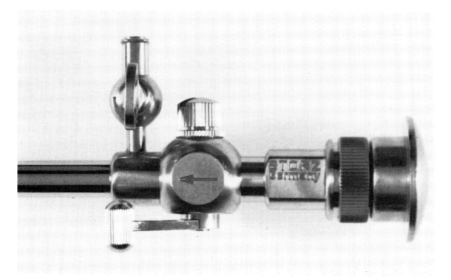

Fig. 1.7b Close-up of examining trocar and cannula with rotating valve and gas inflow stopcock below. The rotating valve is opened during insertion of the telescope. This rotating valve is simpler to use and to maintain than the trapdoor or trumpet valves.

injury to the internal organs. There are three lengths available: a short one for paediatrics, the standard size (length 100 mm) and a longer type (120 mm) for obese abdominal walls. The standard length is preferable in most instances.

The examining trocar and cannula

There are various sizes and types available. We prefer the medium size variety, with an outside diameter of 7 mm. The rotational valve system is easier to handle and maintain than a trap-door or trumpet valve type. In the latter type the seal, during introduction of the pre-warmed telescope, is a gasket which has to be properly positioned. There are two types of sharp trocar: a round conical shape and one with a sharp triangle or pyramid cutting configuration (Figure 1.7a). We prefer the latter type since during the penetration of the abdominal wall achieved by a controlled drilling–pressing action, the resistance of abdominal wall tissue layers is more readily appreciated. Irrespective of its configuration the stylet should be hollow and fitted with a side hole near its tip. The hissing noise of escaping gas through this side hole confirms safe entry into the peritoneal cavity and it is unnecessary to open the valve. It is thus convenient and fast. A stopcock below the valve or trapdoor is necessary to provide gas inflow during the procedure (Figure 1.7b).

The telescope

One should check the sterile telescope first by looking through it from a distance of one inch to make sure it is neither fogged nor damaged before immersing it into the sterile container filled with warm saline. The scope should be pre-warmed above body temperature and dried before insertion. This will avoid fogging of the optical system. A 30° forward oblique direction of view is recommended. The straight forward (0°) direction of view is not suitable for the two-trocar approach, nor is it adequate for thorough examination of the liver and upper abdomen (Figure 1.4).

ACCESSORIES

A fibre-optic cable and sterile tubing for connecting the pneumoperi- toneum needle and later the cannula to the gas insufflator are other essential items. Check the fibre-optic cable from time to time for broken fibres. This can be ascertained with ease by holding one end

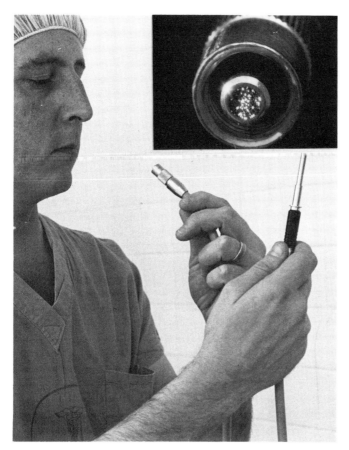

Fig. 1.8 It is worth while examining the light-carrying fibre cable by placing one end in front of a light source and observing the other end. Broken fibres are clearly visible as black dots (see insert). If they predominate, the cable should be replaced.

towards a light and looking at the other end of the fibre bundle (Figure 1.8).

Surgical instruments

A scalpel with a No. 11 blade is used for the stab incisions. A few curved mosquito and larger, Kelly forceps are useful for enlarging the stab incisions. A 10 ml syringe with a 22 gauge needle filled with 1% lignocaine (lidocaine) solution and another 10 ml syringe with 5 ml of saline (for trial aspiration) are required. One pair of scissors and two Babcock or Allis tissue-holding forceps are required to secure the

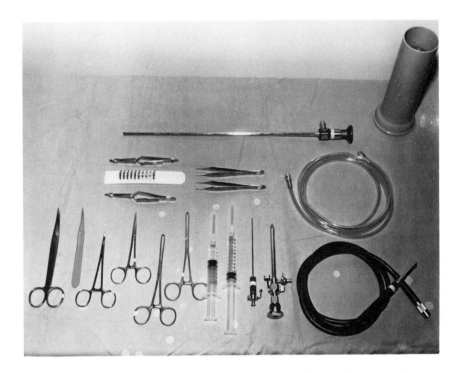

Fig. 1.9 The examining set with some accessories. Top: telescope and container filled with warm saline (prewarmer). Below the telescope: skin clips with appliers; tissue-holding forceps; pneumoperitoneum needle connecting tube. Bottom row: Mayo scissors; scalpel with No. 11 blade; straight and curved haemostats; Allis tissue-holding forceps; syringe with 5 ml of saline; syringe with 10 ml of lignocaine; pneumoperitoneum needle; examining trocar; fibre-optic cable.

gas-carrying tube and the fibre-optic cable to the drapes (Figure 1.9). The use of sharp towel clips for this purpose should be avoided since they may puncture the tubing.

Special accessories

The desufflation key

This is inserted into the trocar when it incorporates a trapdoor system, to allow the gas to escape quickly from the abdominal cavity at the end of the procedure (Figure 1.10).

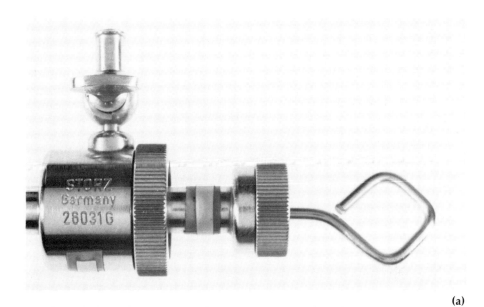

(a)

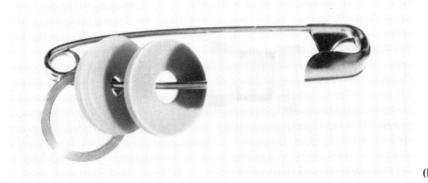

(b)

Fig. 1.10a   If the trocar has a trapdoor valve system a desufflation key has to be inserted at the completion of the procedure to facilitate the removal of gas from the abdominal cavity.   **Fig. 1.10b** A selection of sterile spare parts, such as gaskets, washers and rubber plugs, should be available. There is nothing more frustrating than to have to prolong the procedure unnecessarily because of missing or malfunctioning parts.

Spare parts

A selection of different sized gaskets, washers, rubber plugs and metal rings held on a safety pin (Figure 1.10) should be available on the sterile trolley, preventing unnecessary delays during the examination, since they are easy to drop and lose at the start of the procedure.

Teaching attachment

It is advantageous that the assistant or the nurse has the opportunity to see the pathology. If the procedure is additionally a therapeutic one, requiring the introduction of further instruments, visual control by both the surgeon and the assistant results in much better coordination and greatly facilitates the procedure. A teaching attachment is in essence a beam splitter which doubles the visual image, one going to the operator, the other to the second observer. After adjusting the light output to maximum, a good examining light source can cope with the increased light loss but in case of a dim image a higher intensity light is required. For routine work a rigid teaching attachment is sufficient (Figure 1.11).

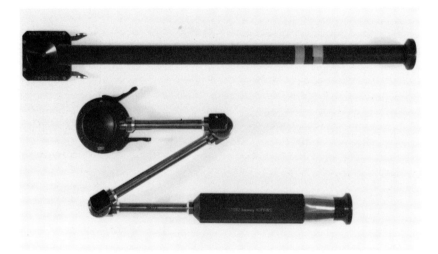

Fig. 1.11 Teaching attachments. Top: the straight type, which is economic and useful. It can be sterilized. Bottom: articulated optical arm with a dual beam-splitter. It can be used as a teaching attachment. For photographic documentation the 90/10% beam-splitter provides maximum image transmission to the camera which is coupled to the viewing end.

There is a more sophisticated teaching attachment available which consists of an articulated optical arm. It has several advantages. Owing to the articulation it is more convenient to use during certain manoeuvres and furthermore it permits photographic documentation since it incorporates a dual beam-splitter (50/50% and 90/10%). The brightness to one side can thus be increased if the splitting ratio is changed to 90/10%: 10% goes to the examiner's eye and 90% to the camera (Figure 2.11). This is an important facility when photography or video recording is required (see Chapter 2).

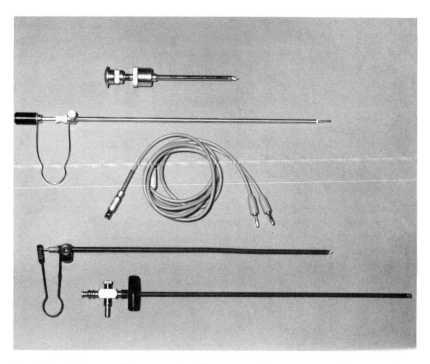

Fig. 1.12   Other sterile accessories. From top to bottom: second (accessory) trocar; bipolar coagulation forceps; high-frequency connecting cable; insulated grasping forceps; insulated suction–coagulation cannula.

Other sterile accessories (Figure 1.12)

1   A *sterile-water container* is available with a built-in lead bottom which minimizes accidental spillage. This is filled with warm, sterile saline. The telescope is inserted for a few minutes and is pre-warmed to above body temperature. It is removed, quickly dried and inserted into the trocar. This will avoid fogging during insertion. Following insertion the telescope cools down to the body temperature.

2   *Second (accessory) trocar* with a stylet. This has an outside diameter of 4 mm. This type of trocar is important for the examination of the upper abdomen. Essentially it is simply a smaller version of the larger trocar.

3   A variety of *biopsy instruments* are required, according to the type and the location of the lesion. There are two types of biopsy forceps: one with a pointed end and the other with punch cutting jaws (Figure 1.13).

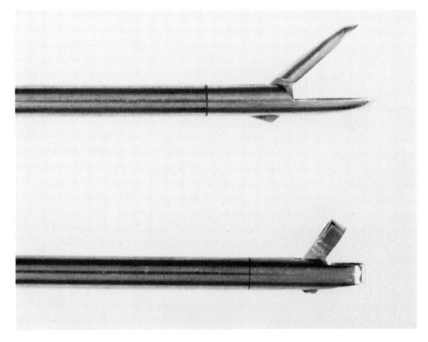

Fig. 1.13 Biopsy forceps. Top: pointed jaws; bottom: punch cutting jaws.

4 *Insulated suction–coagulation–palpation probe.*
5 *Insulated grasping forceps.*
6 *Tru-cut biopsy needle (longer length) or long-shaft Menghini needle.*
7 *High-frequency cable* to connect insulated instruments with the electrosurgical unit.

Non-sterile accessories for laparoscopy

1 *Light source* with spare bulb.
2 *Gas insufflator.* This must be tested before use. A spare gas cylinder should be available.

MAINTENANCE

A well trained operating theatre technician or nurse is essential to ensure that the instruments are maintained in good functioning order until they require replacement. There is nothing more frustrating than to discover after the procedure has started that the optic is foggy or that some important accessories are missing or broken. Having

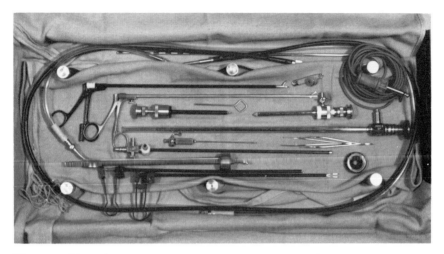

Fig. 1.14   Keep the entire set in one container. It is easier for the nurse and parts are less likely to be mislaid, which can happen if some of them are sterilized or packaged separately.

constantly changing personnel involved in looking after and handling the equipment escalates the frequency and overall cost of repairs. Laparoscopic equipment should not be handled by *any* nurse or operating theatre technician. Instead *one adequately trained* individual should be assigned to this task. The equipment should if possible be used by one operating team. After use the instruments must be meticulously cleaned, disassembled, dried and packed. The entire set should be kept together in one container (Figure 1.14) since this minimizes the risk of losing parts.

STERILIZATION

We prefer gas sterilization because it is a very efficient bactericidal technique and does not damage the instruments. In addition it is convenient since every item is in place after sterilization. If the unit has only one set the instruments can be soaked in Cidex (glutaraldehyde) if they are required for a consecutive examination. With chemical sterilization the instruments must be disassembled, cleaned, soaked and then transferred to a rinsing basin etc.

The method of sterilization must be tailored to the facilities of the hospital, case load and nursing pattern. We do not recommend steam autoclaving as it decreases the lifetime of the equipment. Many manufacturers claim that the optics will withstand this 'insult' provided they are allowed to cool slowly. In practice we have found that the steps described (slow cooling, separate wrapping, etc.) are often overlooked and thus lead to damage of the optics. Although accessories can be autoclaved, this type of sterilization tends to damage the gaskets, which must then be changed more frequently. Laparoscopic instruments should not be flash autoclaved together with surgical hand instruments.

REFERENCES

1   Hopkins, H.H. (1976) Optical principles of the endoscope. (Chapter 1) In *Endoscopy, Berci, G. (ed.)* pp.3–27. New York: Appleton-Century-Crofts.
2   Berci, G. (1976) Instrumentation: rigid endoscopes. (Chapter 5) In *Endoscopy, Berci, G. (ed.)* pp.74–113. New York: Appleton-Century-Crofts.

2

Documentation for Laparoscopy

Margaret Paz-Partlow

INTRODUCTION

A permanent record of an endoscopic procedure is not only desirable but necessary. It allows the physician an opportunity to review any unusual findings. Macroscopic appearance can be compared with histology and computed tomographic scans.[1] The results can be studied in concert with associates for an unlimited period of time without further demands on the patient. A lesion which may have been overlooked at the time of examination can be discovered during subsequent reviews and discussions. A file of endoscopic slides has become invaluable for teaching both postgraduates and undergraduates. Prints made from the slides can be inserted into the patient's chart/records, and also relayed to the referring physician for his or her files (Figure 2.1).[2] A permanent record is especially valuable during the follow-up period for objective comparison of a lesion's progress or regression.

The history of endoscopic photodocumentation dates back to Nitze, who in 1893 developed the first photocystoscope (Figure 2.2).[3] By the turn of the century, he had compiled the first atlas of bladder anatomy and pathology. A major advance was made in 1940 by Holinger, who produced the first endoscopic colour photographs of the bronchial tree.[4] In 1955 Calame introduced a sterilized flash bulb into the abdominal cavity.[5] During the early 1960s Lent and Lindner developed an intracorporeal flash.[6,7] The technical results were quite satisfactory, since the light source was near the object, and the colour temperature of the flash discharge was compatible with 'daylight' film emulsions. The unusually large diameter of the cannula necessary to accommodate the flash was a problem, however. The direction of illumination was another disadvantage, as the light was directed laterally, whereas the optic's direction of view was forward-oblique (Figure 2.3), making it difficult to illuminate long object distances.[8] Finally, its major disadvantage was that of safety. While this system was extremely popular in Europe, its use has been discontinued for some years.

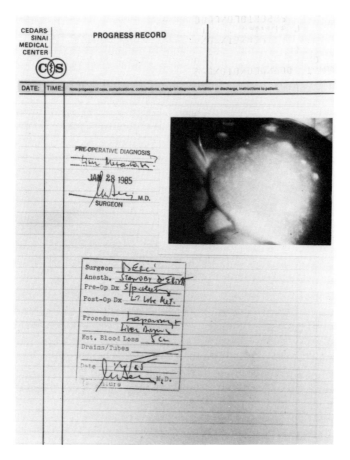

Fig. 2.1 A Polaroid print accompanies and supports the written findings to be inserted in the patient's chart. (Metastatic lesions in the left lobe of the liver.)

GENERAL PRINCIPLES

This leads us to alternative solutions, and the primary problem – illumination. Enough light must be transmitted to the subject and then back to the film plane to ensure adequate exposure. Using both flash and continuous light sources and various endoscopes, we have conducted comparative photometric measurements showing the progressive light loss from the source through the fibre-optic cable and the examining fibres of the endoscope to equal object distances. The output light intensity of a continuous source when passed through a standard 6 ft (1.8 m) fibre cable is reduced by roughly

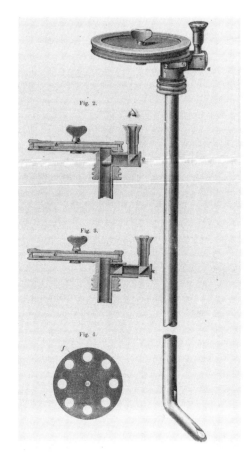

Fig. 2.2 Engraving of Nitze's first photocystoscope; note the disk containing several round coated glass plates. This disc was rotated after each exposure. Using this system, the first atlas of lesions in the urinary bladder was published before the turn of the century.

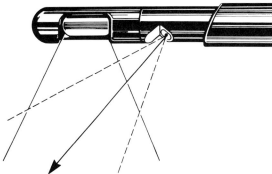

Fig. 2.3 The Lent–Lindner intracorporeal flash globe produced high-intensity illumination, but was not coaxial with the telescope's forward-oblique viewing angle. The strobe discharge failed to match the telescopic angle of view. It was therefore difficult to illuminate longer object distances seen.

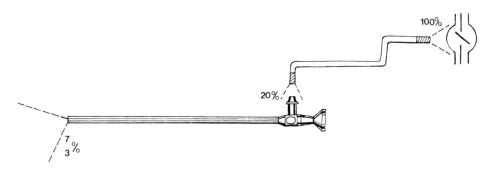

Fig. 2.4   This diagram demonstrates the measured flash light dissipation through intervening systems. Considering the source as 100%, only 20% reaches the endoscope, and only 3–7% reaches the final target.

70–80% (Figure 1.3).[9] The telescope's examining fibres further reduce the final output to approx. 3–7%. Roughly the same proportions of light are lost when a flash tube is used (Figure 2.4). It is difficult to condense a flash discharge onto the small entrance diameter (4 mm) of a fibre bundle, so much of the flash output is lost.[10] Another unavoidable loss results from the 'mismatch' between the individual fibres of the cable and telescope bundles. Light emerging from the core of the first bundle's fibre and falling on the claddings or in the interspaces between the fibres of the second bundle is not trapped and is not transmitted (Figure 2.5).[11]

   Glass fibres are not the only possible means of light transmission. Also available is a fluid cable, which transmits 20% more light than a

Fig. 2.5   The 'mismatch' phenomenon: if a light- (or image-)carrying fibre bundle (F) is connected to another fibre bundle (C), the individual fibres (10–30 μm in diameter) are not optically aligned; therefore, only the overlapping areas (the shaded area on the lower drawing) will transmit light or image, resulting in significant light loss.

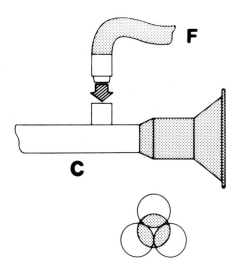

standard 6 ft fibre-optic cable. In addition, the yellowish tint or compression in the red spectral range seen in glass fibre bundles is not apparent thanks to the fluid cable's ability to transmit more light in the blue range.[12]

STILL PHOTOGRAPHY

In an effort to keep the instrumentation as small as possible, one approach has been taken which bypasses entirely the light absorption of the cable and examining bundles and permits still photography with a standard laparoscope. This system couples a 4 mm quartz glass rod directly to an external flash tube and provides the greatest possible illumination (Figure 2.6).[13] However, it does require a third cannula, through which to insert the quartz rod, and more sophisticated manipulative skills in directing it towards the site to be

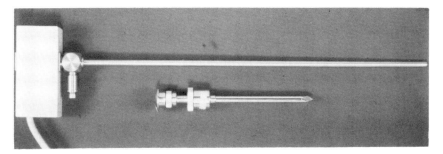

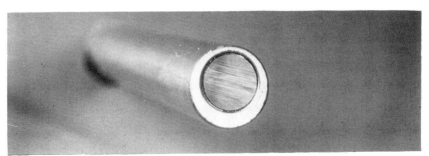

Fig. 2.6 Top: the quartz glass rod with sealed flash globe and trocar. This system provides the greatest illumination, but requires a third puncture and more skill from the operator or assistant to keep the light aimed constantly on the subject. Bottom: quartz rod surrounded by light-carrying (aiming) fibres. The system could be gas sterilized only.

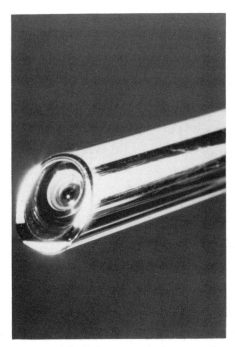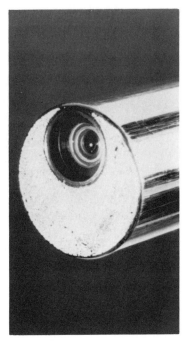

Fig. 2.7   The light transmission area of a standard laparoscope's examining bundles (seen on the left) is significantly less than that of the photolaparoscope (pictured on the right).

photographed. Quartz glass is an excellent transmitter and is better than glass fibres. The large exit angle of this quartz rod permits wide areas to be covered with high-intensity light.

However, the principal approach to increasing illumination for documentation has been the design of a larger telescope incorporating more fibres. The photolaparoscope transmits more light than the examining laparoscope (Figure 2.7). The larger laparoscope requires a larger cannula to be used (Figure 2.8). The abdominal wall is more easily penetrated with the smaller than with the larger trocar,[14] and the operator must manipulate more cautiously when using the larger trocar to avoid possible injury to abdominal organs.

The light source

Earlier quartz glass xenon globes were encased in heavy armour plating and required cumbersome, expensive power supplies and ignition circuits.[15] Efficient continuous high-intensity illumination was introduced ten years ago with an explosion-proof xenon globe

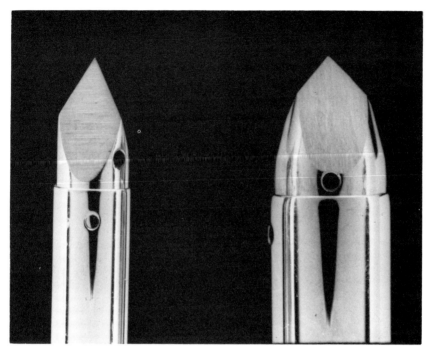

Fig. 2.8 The examining trocar (7 mm) on the left, compared with the filming trocar (11 mm) on the right. In the most recent photolaparoscopes the trocar diameter has been reduced to 9 mm (not pictured).

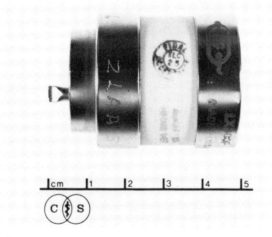

Fig. 2.9 This ceramic-encased xenon globe is the basis of the modern high intensity light source.

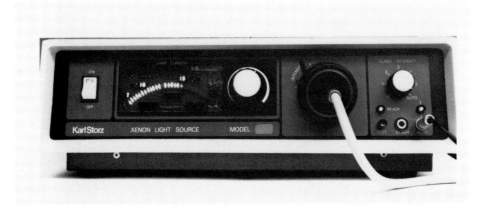

Fig. 2.10   The universal light unit generates both the continuous high-intensity light necessary for television and a flash discharge for 35 mm still photography. The unit can be made compatible with a variety of SLR cameras, whose built-in meters will regulate the flash duration. It is also equipped with an automatic light control for television, maintaining an even level of illumination once it has been set and thus avoiding 'blooming'.

encased in a ceramic housing (Figure 2.9). Owing to the loss in light transmission, even high-intensity continuous light sources do not provide adequate illumination for still photography: long exposure times are required and there is a consequent risk of blurring. A recent electronic power source (Figure 2.10) permits this same globe to be discharged in short flashes providing twice the output of traditional strobe illumination. The duration of the flash may be controlled by the automatic metering system of any modern 35 mm single lens reflex camera. This innovation permits use of a single universal light source for all still photography, cinematography and television applications, since it can be operated in either continuous or stroboscopic mode.

The higher output of this pulsed xenon unit permits interposition of an articulated optical arm between the telescope and the camera. The articulated arm transmits, via rod lenses and prisms, an optical image superior in resolution and brightness to images produced by flexible teaching attachments. The surgeon's eyepiece is equipped with a dual beam-splitter which may be set at 50:50 for simultaneous co-observation, then switched to 90:10 ratio during photography; 90% of the light is then transmitted to the camera (Figure 2.11). The arm may be covered with a sterile sleeve during laparoscopy. Use of this articulated optical arm permits remote placement of the camera, which considerably facilitates manipulation, since the surgeon need

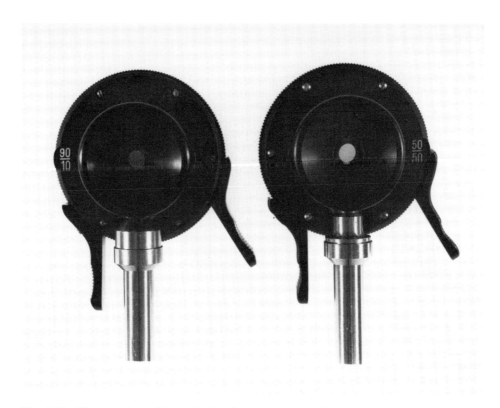

Fig. 2.11 The eyepiece of the articulated arm with its dual beam-splitter – 50/50% for observation and teaching and 90/10% for documentation, with most of the light transmitted to the camera, while still allowing the operator to view the procedure.

not contend with the motorized camera's unwieldy size, weight and extension. The exposure is made either by the circulating nurse or by the surgeon, using a foot control (Figure 2.12). Correct exposure of a medium- to high-speed (200–400 ASA) film is automatically controlled by the through-the-lens metering system. A relatively short recycling time (1–2 sec) permits several exposures to be made without significantly extending operating time.

We have tested both the Kodak and 3M 1000 ASA emulsions, using the pulsed xenon source, a fluid cable and direct attachment to a standard examining laparoscope. While it is possible to achieve adequately exposed photographs in this manner, both resolution and colour display are poor because of the larger grain structure and red spectral compression of the films.

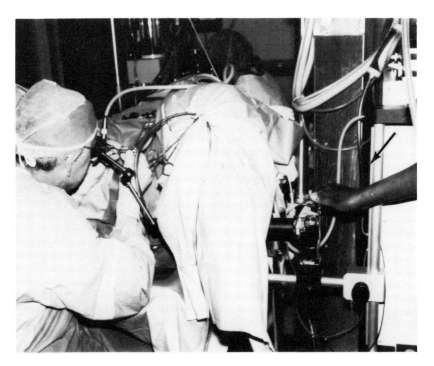

Fig. 2.12 The beam-splitter is attached to a cystoscope. The camera is operated by the circulating nurse (arrowed) or by the surgeon via a footswitch.

16 mm CINEMATOGRAPHY

The universal light unit mentioned above also provides the continuous high-intensity illumination necessary for cinematography. This xenon source provides a higher light density than halogen examining sources. It produces a higher colour temperature (around 5000–6000 kelvin) than the 3200 kelvin typical of standard examining sources. This increase in the blue range of the spectrum makes the light much closer to sunlight and enables generally 'faster', or more sensitive 'daylight' films to be used.

Using a high-intensity light source in conjunction with the photolaparoscope's greater number of light-conducting fibres, one must remember that *more light also means more heat*. When operating at maximum output the heat generated at the working tip of the photolaparoscope is considerable. One must be careful not to cause burn injuries by allowing contact with underlying organs.

Our standard 16 mm camera is the Beaulieu, coupled with a 30 mm C-mount lens fitted with a quick adapter. It is the lightest 16 mm camera available commercially, although its weight (2.2 kg/4.8 lb) still creates problems in camera attachment and manoeuvrability. Efforts were made to produce a lighter, smaller endo-cine camera, but the manufacturing problems proved insoluble, and the camera never advanced beyond prototype status.[16]

Kodak has phased out all of its 16 mm high-speed reversal filmstock except Video News Film (125–400 ASA). This film's coarser grain structure and colour compression towards the reds results in poorer overall reproduction. These deficiencies, coupled with film stock and processing costs, along with laboratory processing delays, mean that cinematography is being rapidly supplanted by improved video techniques.

TELEVISION

The first endo-television camera was reported in 1962,[17] with further refinements in the 1970s.[18] Televised endoscopic procedures have become increasingly favoured for the following reasons:

1 The image can be viewed *immediately*.
2 It can be seen by *several observers simultaneously*.
3 The operator may view an *enlarged image*.
4 It is seen *binocularly* from a *convenient distance*.
5 A *permanent recording* of the findings can be made and reviewed at leisure.

These advantages were previously offset by the inherently inferior image quality of the video systems as compared with photoemulsive resolution. However, recent developments in television technology have altered this perception. Electronic research and development have produced a camera as small as 25 × 25 × 12 mm (1″ × 1″ × ½″), weighing only 50 g (1.6 oz) (Figure 2.13).[19] The camera's minute size is complemented by such additional features as: *sterilizability* (with bactericidal solution or gas), *extreme light sensitivity* (important with instruments with high light absorption) and *optimal dynamic range in the red spectrum* – all extremely valuable characteristics for endoscopic application.

During clinical testing we have successfully employed this solid-state camera in both gynaecological and upper abdominal laparoscopies with excellent results (Figure 2.14). The universal xenon light source was utilized; the camera was directly attached to a

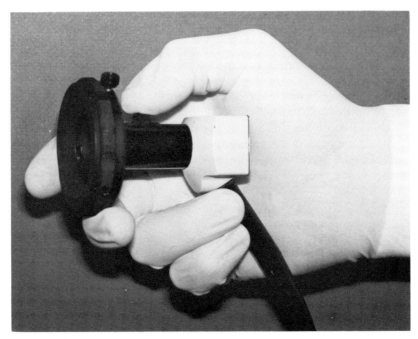

Fig. 2.13   Our present television camera. It is competitive with larger tube cameras in light sensitivity and dynamic colour range. It can be attached to both rigid and flexible endoscopes.

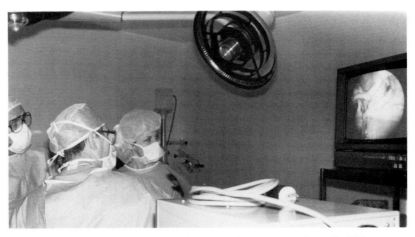

Fig. 2.14   A team of surgeons performing a laparoscopy from the TV screen. The enlarged image, accurate in colour and anatomical detail, enables the operating team to perform more complex procedures with improved coordination, since the operator and assistant can view the organ simultaneously and record interesting findings.

photolaparoscope. The good colour rendition and resolution facilitated the easy recognition of anatomical details, making it possible to complete the examination from the monitor screen. The camera's minimal size and weight did not impede examination, manipulation and biopsies.

One recent innovation in instrumentation promises improvements and simplifications in procedure. Video endoscopes, using a black-and-white sensor chip at the distal tip of a flexible gastro- or colonoscope or a rigid laparoscope, are now available for evaluation. Light conducted by conventional fibre-optic bundles is pulsed through a trichromatic filter system to produce the colour TV image from which the surgeon works. By bypassing the comparatively poorer light transmission and image resolution of the viewing bundles and light absorption of the rigid optics, far more natural colour rendition is achieved. An additional advantage is a freeze-frame capacity, which allows more detailed study of important pathology plus time to expose an instant colour print or 35 mm colour photograph for insertion in the patient's chart. Patient, physician and diagnostic data may be entered with the unit's character generator. Both the written data and endoscopic examination can be concurrently recorded on video tape. As is to be expected in first-generation models, there are mechanical shortcomings yet to be overcome. Nevertheless, video endoscopes augur the future of endoscopic documentation.

CONCLUSIONS

Photodocumentation and simultaneous display of laparoscopic findings are of great value and importance if the surgeon has a large case load or an active teaching programme. Selection of the particular documentation technique according to individual and institutional needs is critical.

Generally, both cinematography and television display are possible for those interested in using them, as is the simpler and more economical option of 35 mm still photography. Continuing research and development have produced a universal light generator capable of both the high intensity continuous illumination required for cine and video applications and the pulsed flash generation needed for still photography. This light source used in conjunction with an articulated optical arm permits remote camera placement, minimizing interference with the examination procedure.

Reduced availability of suitable film emulsions for endoscopic cinematography, coupled with time/cost factors and the increasing availability of smaller, more sensitive and spectrally accurate television cameras, point towards a decreasing role for 16 mm film in laparoscopic documentation. Endoscopic imaging may well be in a period of transition that will culminate in instruments that carry the imaging sensor directly into the body cavity. The performance of existing prototypes suggests that within a matter of years present optical transmission systems may be superseded by the electronic (video) laparoscope.

REFERENCES

1   Berci, G., Merei, F. & Fleischer, J. (1964) Endoscopy and documentation. *Bulletin of Gastrointestinal Endoscopy, 10:* 3.
2   Berci, G., Hasler, G., & Helmuth, J.G. (1976) Permanent film records. In *Endoscopy*, Berci, G. (ed.) New York: Appleton-Century-Crofts.
3   Nitze, M. (1893) Zur Photography der menschlichen Harnrohre. *Berl. med. Wschr. 31:* 744.
4   Holinger, P.H. & Brubaker, J.D. (1941) The larynx, bronchi, and esophagus in Kodachrome. *J. biol. photogr. Ass. 10:* 83.
5   Calame, A. (1956) Laparoscopic photography. *Med. biol. Illust. 6:* 148.
6   Lent, H. (1962) Die Entwicklung der Photolaparoskopie mit dem Electronblitz. *Acta Hepato-splenol. 9:* 195.
7   Lindner, H. (1965) Peritoneoscopic photography with intra-abdominal flash. *Med. biol. Illust. 15:* 146.
8   Berci, G. & Jensen, D. (1982) Laparoscopy for the hepatologist and general surgeon. *Acta Endoscopia 12:* 3.
9   Olsen, V. (1976) Light sources. In *Endoscopy*, Berci, G. (ed.) New York: Appleton-Century-Crofts.
10 Berci, G., Hasler, G., & Helmuth, J.G. (1976) Permanent film records. In *Endoscopy*, Berci, G. (ed.) New York: Appleton-Century-Crofts.
11 Hopkins, H.H. (1976) Physics of the fiberoptic endoscope. In *Endoscopy*, Berci, G. (ed.) New York: Appleton-Century-Crofts.
12 Mautner, W.J. (1976) High energy wave guides. In *Endoscopy*, Berci, G. (ed.) New York: Appleton-Century-Crofts.
13 Jensen, D. & Berci, G. (1981) Laparoscopy: advances in biopsy and recording techniques. *Gastrointestinal Endoscopy, 27:* 150.
14 Berci, G., Adler, D., Brooks, P. et al. (1973) The importance of instrumentation and documentation in gynecological laparoscopy. *J. repro. Med. 10:* 6.
15 Olsen, V. (1976) Light sources. In *Endoscopy*, Berci, G. (ed.) New York: Appleton-Century-Crofts.
16 Berci, G. (1976) Techniques for improving illumination and recording in endoscopy. *Optics and Laser Technology, 2:* 31.
17 Berci, G. & Davids, J. (1962) Endoscopy and television. *Br. med. J. i:* 1610.
18 Berci, G. & Urban, J.C. (1972) Miniature black and white TV camera for endoscopy and other medical applications. *Bio-Med. Engng, 7:* 116.
19 Berci, G., Schulman, A.G., Morgenstern, L. et al. (1985) TV choledochoscopy. *Surgery Gynec. Obstet. 160:* 176.

3
Indications and Contraindications for Diagnostic Laparoscopy

Indications	Contraindications – absolute and relative
Liver disease	Mechanical or paralytic ileus
Suspected liver tumours	Blood dyscrasias and coagulopathies
Suspected metastases	General peritonitis
Palpable abdominal mass	Obesity
Ascites of unknown origin	Large hiatus hernia
Tumour staging	Irreducible external hernia
Second look	Abdominal wall sepsis
Chronic pain of unknown origin	Severe cardiovascular or respiratory disease
Abdominal diagnostic dilemmas	
Fever of unknown origin	

INDICATIONS

Liver disease. Both liver lobes can be seen, the extent of the disease assessed and important features discovered – for example, distended veins on the parietal peritoneum and on the round or falciform ligament, indicating portal hypertension etc. In the hands of an experienced endoscopist laparoscopic liver biopsy is safer than the blind percutaneous technique since bleeding can be controlled by diathermy. Furthermore, the site of the biopsy can be selected and more accurate information obtained than from a blind tissue sample, especially in the presence of focal disease.[1,2]

The majority of percutaneous liver biopsies are performed with a Tru-cut needle or Menghini aspiration technique and both may yield unsatisfactory or fragmented minute particles. With a visually aimed process the area under suspicion can be selected, the target approached with precision and an adequate core of tissue retrieved.

Suspected liver tumours. In the Western hemisphere primary hepatic tumours usually arise on a background of cirrhosis. Much less commonly they originate in a previously normal liver. Cirrhomimetic cases are often heralded by a rapid deterioration of the clinical picture, which should alert the attending clinician. The differentiation between the two forms of the disease, which can be easily made by laparoscopy, is important since the presence of cirrhosis often precludes lobectomy and is a contraindication to trisegmentectomy. As well as detecting cirrhosis, laparoscopy is invaluable in assessing the extent of the disease, particularly in determining whether the tumour involves one or both lobes and whether it is multicentric.

Suspected metastases. Laparoscopy is more accurate than a needle aspiration under CT or ultrasonic guidance. Aspiration cytology is inferior to tissue samples taken by forceps or needle core biopsy. Laparoscopy with target biopsy allows the clinician to establish the presence of advanced disease and obtain a biopsy for histological confirmation.

Palpable mass. Not infrequently the 'clinically enlarged liver' or 'hepatic mass' is found to be normal at laparoscopy, the pathology being extrahepatic but adjacent to the liver. In particular, high protruding (retroperitoneal) tumours and omental masses involving jejunum or transverse colon are often misdiagnosed as hepatomegaly. With large intra-abdominal tumours, the veins on the surface of the lesion are engorged and easily damaged by blind puncture: severe bleeding ensues. Laparoscopic inspection and target biopsy avoids this complication. Again, a higher diagnostic yield is obtained and assessment of the extent of the disease can be achieved.

Ascites of unknown origin. When the cause of the ascites remains uncertain despite routine non-invasive investigation, laparoscopy is the method of choice to confirm the diagnosis. Laparoscopy with target biopsy is invaluable in the diagnosis of abdominal tuberculosis and primary and secondary peritoneal tumours. A percutaneous liver biopsy may be difficult or impossible to perform in a patient with gross ascites and a failed blind biopsy may be an indication for laparoscopy.

Staging. In patients with known primary tumours a laparoscopy prior to laparotomy can yield information which may alter the surgical approach and in some cases obviate the necessity for laparotomy.[3,4]

Second look. Laparoscopy provides an alternative to laparotomy in the detection of recurrent disease after surgical extirpation and in assessing the effect of adjuvant radio/chemotherapy for gastrointestinal, pancreatic and hepatobiliary cancer.

Chronic pain of unknown origin. The procedure is useful in cases where investigations have failed to elucidate the cause of pain. In a consecutive prospective series of patients with undiagnosed abdominal pain submitted to laparoscopy we have encountered significant pathology including previously unsuspected cancer in 30%.[5]

Abdominal diagnostic dilemmas. In the elderly patient, it is difficult sometimes to obtain an accurate history. Furthermore, the physical signs in the abdomen can be misleading. Laboratory data, despite the presence of an inflammatory or other organic disease, can be non-contributory. In many of these cases laparoscopy can assist in discovering acute pathology, such as an inflamed appendix and mesenteric vascular insufficiency. In young females, the differential diagnosis of right lower quadrant tenderness (appendicitis *vs.* pelvic inflammatory disease) can be obtained. It is also helpful in children with suspected appendicitis.[6]

Fever of unknown origin. The inspection of the abdominal cavity, guided biopsy of suspected areas and inspection of the spleen can assist diagnosis in patients with pyrexia of unknown origin. Enlarged lymph nodes, matted intestinal loops, omental mass, free fluid in paracolic gutters, hyperaemic oedematous intestine etc. may prove diagnostic and indicate the need for surgical intervention.

CONTRAINDICATIONS

Mechanical or paralytic ileus. A patient with a distended abdomen due to air- or air–fluid-filled intestinal loops displayed on the X-ray film should never be submitted to laparoscopy.

Blood dyscrasias and coagulopathies. Correctable coagulation disorders do not constitute a contraindication, but they do require prior replacement therapy. Improvement after treatment should be confirmed before the procedure is performed. If the abnormal coagulation state proves refractory, then laparoscopy should be avoided. Each case has to be assessed individually. Aspirin abusers, including those on prescribed high doses, or addicts need special attention.

General peritonitis. If the clinical picture is obvious, the surgeon should resort to laparotomy. Localized peritonitis, on the other hand, is not a contraindication and the laparoscopic findings may alter the surgical approach.

Obesity. In case of extreme morbid obesity, the examination should not be performed because the lengths of the pneumoperitoneum needle and trocar may not exceed the thickness of the abdominal wall. In addition laparoscopic inspection is difficult and unreliable in the presence of a gross and redundant omentum.

Hiatus hernia. Large hiatus hernia can result in a pneumomediastinum after laparoscopy and is usually considered to be a contraindication, though with CO_2 insufflation the procedure can be performed without any adverse effects.

Cardio-respiratory disease. Decompensated cardiac disease, cardiac disease accompanied by conduction defects and recent myocardial infarction (within three months) are contraindications to laparoscopy but compensated cardiac disease and angina are not. Severe obstructive respiratory disease ($FEV_1 < 1.0$ litre) is also a contraindication.

Previous abdominal surgery. This is not a contraindication. However, the site of puncture has to be chosen carefully (for details see Chapter 5).

Irreducible external hernia. There is a risk of ischaemia of the hernial contents of an external hernia when the intraperitoneal pressure is increased by the artificial pneumoperitoneum. For this reason an irreducible external hernia of any type is considered a contraindication to laparoscopy.

Abdominal wall sepsis. This is an absolute contraindication because of the risk of peritoneal infection.

REFERENCES

1   Cuschieri, A. (1975) Value of laparoscopy in hepatobiliary disease. *Ann. R. Coll. Surg.* 57: 33–38.
2   Berci, G. (1976) Laparoscopy in general surgery. In *Endoscopy*, Berci, G. (ed.) pp. 382–401. New York: Appleton-Century-Crofts.
3   Cuschieri, A. (1980) Laparoscopy in general surgery and gastroenterology. *Hosp. Med.* 24: 252–258.

4   Shandall, A. & Johnson, C. (1985) Laparoscopy or scanning in oesophageal carcinoma. *Br. J. Surg. 72:* 449–451.
5   Wood, R.A.B. & Cuschieri, A. (1979) Laparoscopy for chronic abdominal pain. *Br. J. Surg. 60:* 900.
6   Gans, S.L. & Berci, G. (1973) Peritoneoscopy in infants and children. *J. pediat. Surg. 8:* 399–405.

4
Anaesthesia

Adequate anaesthesia and analgesia are essential for the safety of a laparoscopic procedure. There is some resistance among anaesthetists to local anaesthesia for the procedure since general anaesthesia with endotracheal intubation and controlled ventilation is considered safer should cardio-respiratory complications occur during the procedure. This belief is based more on lack of experience than fact. A pneumoperitoneum can be created safely under local anaesthesia provided that the patient is adequately sedated throughout the procedure. For successful laparoscopy under local anaesthesia, intravenous medication is the key factor. The patient has to be *somnolent but responsive*, such that dull pressure can be felt, but under no circumstances should pain be experienced. A well premedicated patient will not recall the procedure.

Laparoscopy can be performed under *general, regional* or *local anaesthesia*. Each approach has its advantages, limitations and complications. Local anaesthesia carries the least morbidity and is the routine in most centres. In practice the type of anaesthesia is influenced by the patient's condition, the disease and the estimated risk factors. In young fit patients, for example, females undergoing gynaecological laparoscopy, general anaesthesia is the preferred method and does not impose any increased risk.

It is very important for the operator to develop good communication and understanding with the anaesthetist. Adequate preoperative assessment of the patient and the disease minimizes the risk. The necessary measures should be undertaken to correct metabolic and haematological abnormalities. These include hypokalaemia, hyponatraemia, hyperglycaemia, azotaemia, anaemia and coagulation defects. All the required laboratory data should be available, including blood grouping and testing for the hepatitis B antigen. Elderly patients should have an electrocardiogram and chest X-ray.

REGIONAL ANAESTHESIA

Spinal anaesthesia is reported enthusiastically for gynaecological procedures without significant complications.[10] We do not have experience with this type of anaesthesia for this procedure but it seems to us that it is mainly useful for pelvic procedures. Bilateral lower intercostal nerve block has also been used, but it is time-consuming and may be complicated by pneumothorax.

GENERAL ANAESTHESIA

Some centres use general anaesthesia as a routine in all cases. General anaesthesia is advisable in children. Endotracheal anaesthesia with muscular relaxants and controlled ventilation is generally preferred especially in elderly or high-risk cases. General anaesthesia is also preferable for interventional laparoscopy.

Some advocate open anaesthesia, which avoids the post-intubation sore throat and laryngeal sequelae, but this is associated with a risk of inhalation and gastric distension. The latter is circumvented by the passage of a nasogastric tube. Halothane should be avoided or used sparingly in patients with several previous operations and in the presence of liver disease.

LOCAL ANAESTHESIA

The large number of laparoscopic procedures performed under local anaesthesia with intravenous sedation and with minimal morbidity and negligible mortality (0.5–1.0 per thousand) testifies to the feasibility and safety of this method. We prefer to perform laparoscopy under local anaesthesia with an anaesthetist being present to monitor the patient's cardiac and respiratory functions. Intravenous sedation is carried out with Diazemuls (i.v. diazepam in Intralipid) and pethidine. As local anaesthetic we use 1% lignocaine without adrenaline (lidocaine without epinephrine). It is very important that the sites of insertion of the needle, trocar and secondary accessory trocar are infiltrated not only along the line of insertion, but over the entire area of expected movements to avoid this important source of pain: the sensitive parietal peritoneum has to be anaesthetized over an adequate area (Figures 4.1 and 4.2).

It has to be clearly understood by every operator who intends to perform this procedure under local anaesthesia that it can be done in the majority of cases if adequate sedation and analgesia are administered to keep the patient somnolent but responsive. Another important aspect is continuous monitoring. It is preferable to perform the procedure in the operating room. It can be done in a clean endoscopy area as long as monitoring and resuscitation equipment is available.

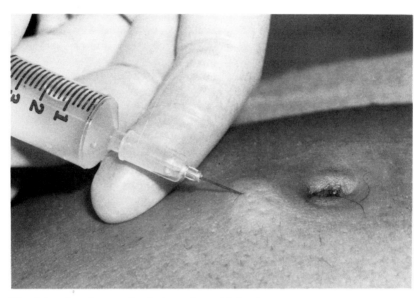

Fig. 4.1a   Local anaesthesia: intradermal injection.

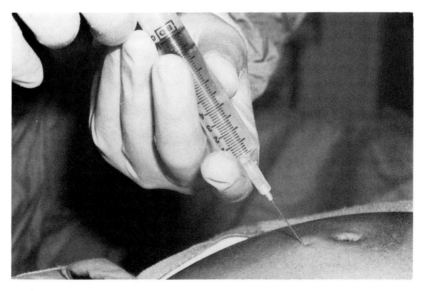

Fig. 4.1b   This is followed by deeper infiltration with 1% lignocaine.

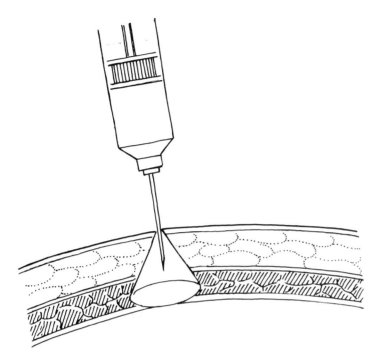

Fig. 4.2   The infiltration of the parieties should cover a cone-shaped block of tissue with the base at the parietal peritoneum in order to block the sensory nerves in this important layer. In this way no painful stimuli are created during the movements of the trocar.

When using local anaesthesia we prefer that the anaesthetist administers the pethidine (meperidine) and Diazemuls slowly via an intravenous line. In elderly patients one should be cautious with Diazemuls but more generous with pethidine. The patient is connected to a blood pressure and pulse monitoring device as well as to an ECG monitor. Patients should have an intravenous line inserted before the procedure.

If a pneumoperitoneum is created with caution, minor changes in blood pressure or pulse (± 10% of the pre-procedure level) can be tolerated well for this short procedure. It is advisable to administer oxygen through the nose or via a mask; this can help to overcome the slight hypercarbia which may develop. Every pneumoperitoneum is unpleasant, because of stretching of the sensitive parietal peritoneum and increased pressure on the diaphragm. Vago-vagal reflexes can occur and increased pressure on the inferior vena cava can reduce the cardiac output. If the patient is adequately medicated, with a proper depth of somnolence, the majority of pain-releasing stimuli or reflexes are eliminated. Cardiac arrhythmias are common. Pressure should not be increased above 20 mmHg (2.7 kPa). If the abdomen is over-distended and arrhythmias occur, these can be immediately reversed by prompt desufflation of the abdominal cavity. A regular heart rhythm will return. At this stage, slow infusion of gas can recommence. Premedication with atropine (0.5 mg) can help to decrease the cardiac irritability caused by vagal stimulation.

In our institution, where 90% of examinations are performed under local anaesthesia with intravenous medication, we have not encountered a single instance of cardiac or respiratory arrest. Those arrhythmias which developed reversed after desufflation. No severe haemodynamic complications of the pneumoperitoneum, such as shock, have been observed.

After the procedure, and irrespective of the type of anaesthesia used, the patient should be observed in a recovery area for 2 hours. If the vital signs are stable, the patient can be transferred back to the ward with strict orders for vital signs to be monitored every half hour for the next four hours; the patient must be kept in bed. The intravenous line should not be removed until the patient is able to tolerate liquids, which is usually 4–6 hours postoperatively.

REFERENCES

1   Lewis, G.B.H. & Prasad, K. (1974) Sodium bicarbonate treatment of ventricular arrhythmias during laparoscopy. *Anesthesiology. 41(4):* 416.
2   Diamant, M., Benumof, J.L. & Saidman, L.J. (1978) Hemodynamics of increased intra-abdominal pressure: interaction with hypovolemia and halothane anesthesia. *Anesthesiology. 48:* 23–27.
3   Diamant, M., Benumof, J.L., Saidman, L.J., Kennedy, J. & Young, P. (1977) Laparoscopic sterilization with local anesthesia: complications and blood-gas changes. *Anesth. Analg. 56 (3):* 335–337.
4   Fishburne, J.I., Fulghum, M.S., Hulka, J.F. & Mercer, J.P. (1974) General anesthesia for outpatient laparoscopy with an objective measure of recovery. *Anesth. Analg. 53(1):* 1–6.
5   Drury, W.L., LaVallee, D.A. & Vacanti, C.J. (1971) Effects of laparoscopic tubal ligation on arterial blood gases. *Anesth. Analg. 50(3):* 349–351.
6   Motew, M., Ivankovich, A.D., Bieniarz, J., Albrecht, R.F., Zahed, B. & Scommegna, A. (1973) Cardiovascular effects and acid–base and blood gas changes during laparoscopy. *Am. J. Obstet. Gynecol. 115(7):* 1002–1012.
7   Scott, D.B. & Julian, D.G. (1972) Observations on cardiac arrhythmias during laparoscopy. *Br. med. J. i:* 411–413.
8   Gordon, N.L.M., Smith, I. & Swapp, G.H. (1972) Cardiac arrhythmias during laparoscopy. *Br. med. J. i:* 625.

9   Utting, J.E. (1972) Cardiac arrhythmias during laparoscopy. *Br. med. J. i:* 566.

10 Alexander, G.D., Noe, F.E. & Brown, E.M. (1969) Anesthesia for pelvic laparoscopy. *Anesth. Analg. 48(1):* 14–18.

11 Sharp, J.R., Pierson, W.P. & Brady III, C.E. (1982) Comparison of CO_2- and N_2O-induced discomfort during peritoneoscopy under local anesthesia. *Gastroenterology, 82:* 453–456.

12 Hodgson, C., McClelland, R.M.A. & Newton, J.R. (1970) Some effects of the peritoneal insufflation of carbon dioxide at laparoscopy. *Anesthesia, 25(3):* 382–390.

13 Peterson, E.P. (1971) Anesthesia for laparoscopy. *Fert. Steril. 22(10):* 695 690.

14 Wheeless Jr, C.R. (1971) Anesthesia for diagnostic and operative laparoscopy. *Fert. Steril. 22(10):* 690–694.

15 Scott, D.B. (1972) Cardiac arrhythmias during laparoscopy. *Br. med. J. ii:* 49–50.

16 Morley, T.R. (1972) Cardiac arrhythmias during laparoscopy. *Br. med. J. ii:* 295–296.

17 Lode, H., Huttemann, U. & Wolff, C.V. (1972) Der Einfluss endoskopischer abdomineller Untersuchungen auf die Atmung. *Respiration, 29:* 61–73.

18 Marshall, R.L., Jebson, P.J.R., Davie, I.T. & Scott, D.B. (1972) Circulatory effects of carbon dioxide insufflation of the peritoneal cavity for laparoscopy. *Br. J. Anaesth. 44:* 680–684.

5

Creation of a Pneumoperitoneum and Trocar Insertion

THE PNEUMOPERITONEUM

The creation of an adequate pneumoperitoneum is the most important step of the entire procedure. The aim is to build up a good protective cushion to ensure the safe introduction of the trocar and good visibility for the examination and subsequent procedures. The majority of complications are results of an inadequate pneumoperitoneum and/or poor technique. These complications can be largely avoided by adequate training and attention to important practical details.

Choice of insufflating agent

In the past room air was used to inflate the abdomen by connecting a Higginson's bulb to the needle. The simplicity of this appealed to many laparoscopists, but the method has major disadvantages which should preclude its use nowadays:

1 Inadvertently introducing air into a vessel can cause air embolism, with a fatal outcome.
2 Without continuous pressure measurement one cannot recognize the accidental insufflation of air into the omentum and mesentery or penetration of hollow viscera.
3 There is a risk of peritoneal infection with contaminated air, especially if this is unfiltered.

Instead either CO_2 or N_2O is used; the relative merits are shown in Table 5.1. CO_2 has the advantage of being non-combustible and allows the concomitant use of electro-coagulation and laser irradiation. It is absorbed in small amounts into the bloodstream but with the correct technique this does not result in any significant acidosis. After the procedure any residual CO_2 is absorbed from the peritoneal cavity within 30 minutes postoperatively. N_2O is absorbed at a slower rate and can be used for the same purposes, except for electrocoagulation. There is some debate as to whether CO_2 irritates the peritoneum more than N_2O when the procedure is performed under local

44

Table 5.1   Comparison of CO_2 and N_2O as insufflating gases

CO_2	N_2O
1 Non-inflammable; does not support combustion	Non-inflammable, but supports combustion
2 Painful	Less painful
3 Causes a fall in pH, Po_2 and serum chloride and a rise in Pco_2	No significant changes
4 Low but definite incidence of cardiac arrhythmias	Cardiac arrhythmias significantly less common than with CO_2
5 Cardiovascular changes persist for a while after desufflation	Cardiovascular changes return to normal soon after desufflation

anaesthesia. In our opinion, the most important factor in the prevention of pain is not the type of gas but adequate analgesia and sedation. If this is achieved the patient will not experience pain and will sustain total amnesia for the event. It is very important to maintain close observation and monitoring during the insufflation phase so that any haemodynamic changes that occur can be immediately recognized and dealt with.

The insufflator

Before the patient's skin is prepared and draped, the insufflation apparatus should be checked. The basic principles apply irrespective of the type of insufflator used (Figure 5.1). One should always ensure

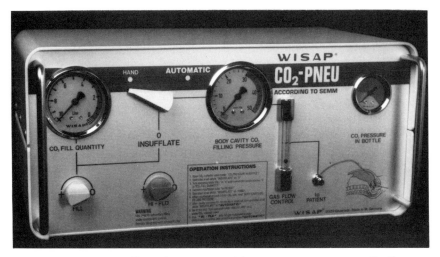

Fig. 5.1 CO_2 gas insufflator for creation of the pneumoperitoneum. Similar units are available for N_2O insufflation.

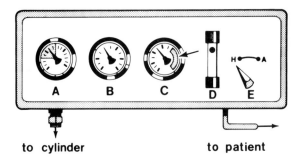

to cylinder   to patient

Fig. 5.2 Diagram of insufflator. *A: cylinder gauge.* If the needle gauge is below the shaded area the gas cylinder should be exchanged. *B: volume gauge.* This indicates the volume in litres instilled into the peritoneal cavity. *C: intra-abdominal pressure gauge.* This measures the resistance of the pneumoperitoneum needle as well. In general the pressure reading after insertion of the Veress needle should be 5–10 mmHg (0.7–1.3 kPa). If the pressure recorded is higher, especially if it goes towards the shaded, high-pressure zone (30–50 mmHg/4.0–6.6 kPa), the needle tip is in the wrong place and the position of the needle should be changed until the pressure drops to 5–10 mmHg. *D: flow-meter. E: switch.* H = hand position: continuous inflow at 50mmHg pressure. A = automatic position: inflow regulated by pressure. In this position, if the pressure rises above 16 mmHg (2.1 kPa) the insufflator shuts off automatically until the pressure falls, when insufflation of the peritoneal cavity restarts.

that enough gas is present in the supply cylinder; this is indicated by a pressure gauge (Figure 5.2 – A). If it is near empty, it is better to change the cylinder before the procedure, than to run out of gas during the procedure. The second dial is the volume gauge (Figure 5.2 – B). The insufflated volume necessary to distend the abdomen varies greatly from patient to patient. It depends on the distensibility of the abdominal wall, obesity, sex and the presence of ascites. Although the average volume necessary is 3–4litres, the exact amount required to achieve an adequate cushion has to be judged for each patient. It is very important to check the abdomen from time to time by percussion, making sure that it is symmetrically tympanic. A tight abdomen is necessary for safe manipulations. However, one should not exceed an intra-abdominal pressure of 20mmHg (2.7 kPa). The pressure gauge (Figure 5.2 – C) is used to monitor the intra-abdominal pressure during the procedure and before insufflation. If the pressure gauge reading exceeds the 10mmHg mark (1.3kPa), this signifies that the needle tip is in a wrong position. The flow meter (Figure 5.2 – D) shows the constant flow of gas into the abdominal cavity. The selector switch (Figure 5.2 – E) has two positions: H, for hand, and A, for automatic. At the start of

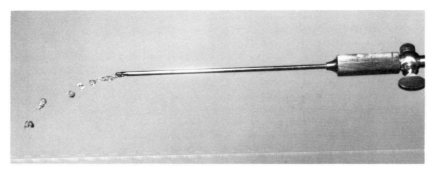

Fig. 5.3   The patency of the pneumoperitoneum is checked by injecting saline through it.

insufflation this switch should be in the H position (continuous flow at 50 mmHg pressure (6.7 kPa)). Flow should not exceed 1–1.2 litres per minute. The equipment should be checked from time to time to ensure that it still conforms to the manufacturers' specifications. If a spirometer is available it can be used to check the flow per minute and peak level.

The pneumoperitoneum needle should be checked to ensure that the spring-loaded stylet is functioning properly and the lumen is patent. This can be achieved by squirting a few millilitres of water through the needle (Figure 5.3).

The normal abdomen

The selection of the insertion site for the pneumoperitoneum needle is very important, especially in the operated abdomen (see pp. 52–54). In the normal non-operated person there is a choice of three safe sites. The most common one is the midline just below the umbilical fold (Figure 5.4). At this stage the abdomen is already prepped and draped and the tubes to the insufflator apparatus and fibre-optic cable are secured to the drapes. The site for the needle insertion is infiltrated generously with local anaesthetic. We use a 1% lignocaine solution without adrenaline (lidocaine without epinephrine). The peritoneum is well innervated and therefore very sensitive. An injection in a straight line of a few millilitres of local anaesthetic is insufficient: the patient will sense pain.

Standard local anaesthetic procedures should be followed. First, a skin or intradermal injection is made, creating the orange peel appearance. The abdominal wall is infiltrated layer by layer, aspirating at each layer to confirm that neither blood vessels nor intestines have been penetrated. A cone-shaped volume of whole

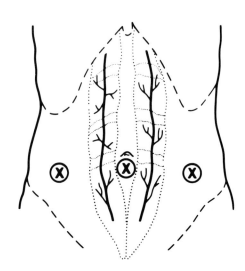

Fig. 5.4 The preferred sites of insertion of the pneumoperitoneum needle in a normal (non-operated) abdomen: below the umbilicus in the midline or in the right or left lower quadrant at the umbilicus– iliac crest line, lateral third. These sites are chosen to avoid injury to the epigastric vessels and their branches.

thickness abdominal wall including the peritoneum is infiltrated to ensure painless manipulations.

After waiting a few minutes to allow the local anaesthetic to take effect a skin stab incision is made, using a No. 11 blade (Figure 5.5). Initially the incision should not be deep, because in a thin abdominal wall these fine-pointed blades can easily damage underlying organs. If a large incision is made, gas will leak around the needle or trocar.

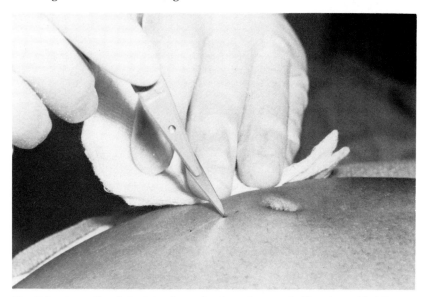

Fig. 5.5 A small stab incision is made after adequate infiltration with 1% lignocaine (lidocaine). Only the skin is incised.

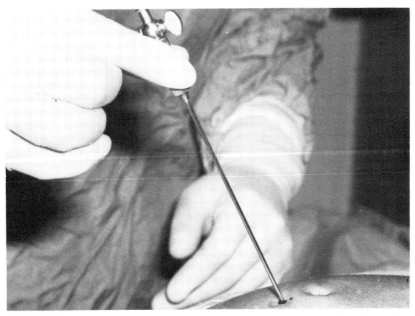

Fig. 5.6 The pneumoperitoneum needle is held by its serrated handle and introduced into the abdominal cavity. An audible click is heard as the spring-loaded blunt stylet jumps into position.

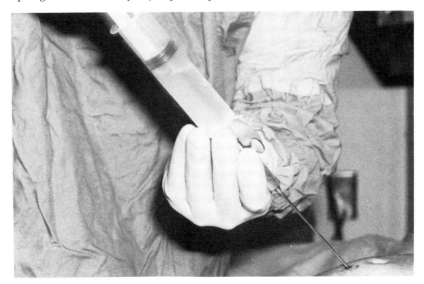

Fig. 5.7 A syringe with saline is attached and aspiration is applied. If blood or yellowish fluid is aspirated the needle position is changed. After aspiration, 1–2 ml of saline is injected to ensure that omentum has not been sucked into the needle side-hole.

The Veress needle is introduced perpendicularly to the abdominal wall (Figure 5.6). The click of the spring-loaded blunt stylet should be felt as it is pushed back into the needle while traversing the various layers. The blunt stylet springs out of the needle with an audible click as it enters the peritoneal cavity. The next step consists of trial aspiration. After attaching a 10 ml syringe filled with 5 ml of saline one should aspirate and inject a few millilitres and then repeat the procedure (Figure 5.7). Aspiration is necessary to ensure the safe position of the needle tip within the peritoneal cavity. Injection of a few millilitres of saline is required to avoid blockage of the stylet side hole by nearby omentum. Many of the reported accidents are preventable if trial aspiration is performed. If blood-stained fluid or frank blood is recovered the needle position should be changed. This entails complete withdrawal of the Veress needle and its reinsertion at a slightly different angle. Thereafter the aspiration should be repeated, and if there is no positive sign (blood or yellowish fluid) the insufflation can be started. The aspiration of blood-stained fluid should not cause concern, but has to be noted and kept in mind before desufflation is carried out. The area under the needle insertion should be scanned with the telescope to confirm that there is no major blood pooling. Aspiration of yellowish fluid indicates that the needle has entered the gastrointestinal lumen. A hole in the bowel of this small size (2 mm) does not warrant surgical intervention, but close observation is required. A nasogastric tube should be inserted and the patient kept on intermittent suction, intravenous fluids and antibiotics for 24–48 hours. After ascertaining that the needle is in the proper position it is connected to the gas insufflator, set for continuous flow.

Once the pneumoperitoneum is completed and the trocar is inserted, the continuous flow must be changed to automatic. This mechanism stops gas inflow when the intra-abdominal pressure exceeds 16 mmHg (2.1 kPa) and re-opens if it falls below this level. This provides a safety measure against over-inflation of the peritoneal cavity. In practice, gas is often lost during the procedure and this leads to impaired vision due to partial collapse of the pneumoperitoneum. Whenever this happens, the circulating nurse is asked to change the switch back to the Hand position, and a careful watch is kept on the intra-abdominal pressure, which should not exceed *20 mmHg (2.7 kPa)*. The nurse and the operator should observe the intra-abdominal pressure gauge and *switch back to the automatic position* as soon as the optimal pneumoperitoneum is re-established.

During insertion of the needle a 'trick of the trade' which is especially useful in obese patients is to ask the patient to lift up his or her head for a few seconds. This increases the tension of the abdominal muscles and minimizes indenting of the muscle layers ahead of the needle/trocar, thereby facilitating penetration of the abdominal wall. The patient should be instructed about this prior to premedication. Lifting of the abdominal wall by the operator is helpful in thin patients, but in slightly obese and in multiparous females the manoeuvre is of little value since only the skin and subcutaneous fat are elevated.

After 1–2 minutes of insufflation the abdominal pressure gauge should move in synchrony with the respiration, indicating a free position of the needle tip in the peritoneal cavity with transmission of pressure waves caused by the movement of the diaphragm. After two minutes, during which time approximately two litres of gas will have been insufflated, it is also advisable to move the serrated handle of the needle in a small circle. This will cause the distal end of the needle to move in a larger radius (Figure 5.8). If the needle tip is in a free area during these circular movements the intra-abdominal pressure will

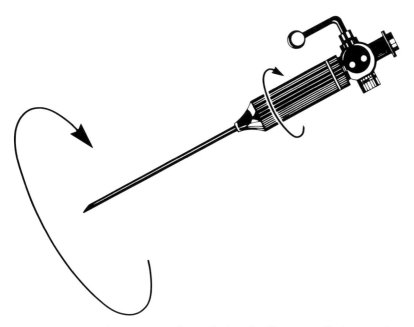

Fig. 5.8 After a few minutes of insufflation the Veress needle is rotated at an angle to the abdominal wall such that the needle tip inside the peritoneal cavity encircles a large area. If this step results in no increase in the abdominal pressure it can be safely assumed that the needle is lying free in the peritoneal cavity. On the other hand, a rise in pressure following this manoeuvre indicates that the needle is in a confined area and repositioning is necessary.

not change. By contrast, if the needle tip hits an organ or is entangled in omentum, or if an omental pouch has been created by the insufflation, this circular movement will cause the pressure to rise. The intra-abdominal pressure gauge is thus a very helpful indicator of the exact position of the needle tip. It is not uncommon for the needle to be inserted within adhesions or to come to lie between the leaves of the mesocolon or mesentery, creating a 'balloon' effect, with increased pressure. Therefore, if the pressure increases rapidly – for instance, if it exceeds 20 mmHg within 1–2 minutes – the insufflation should be stopped and the needle position changed. Often, when this happens, subsequent inspection with the laparoscope of the area below the needle insertion will reveal a foamy appearance of the omentum or mesentery indicating this phenomenon. Sometimes litres of gas can be inadvertently trapped in these areas and render adequate inspection of the abdomen unsatisfactory. This gas will disperse in the retroperitoneum.

It is also important to observe the patient's response to increased intra-abdominal pressure. If the patient starts to move or indicates pain, the insufflation should be interrupted and more intravenous medication administered. The insufflation can be resumed when the patient is more somnolent. ECG monitoring and observation of the vital signs are continued throughout. If cardiovascular changes are observed, desufflation is necessary. However, if the changes reverse, the procedure can recommence.

When the pneumoperitoneum is properly established and the pressure has reached 20 mmHg, palpation reveals a tight abdomen with a symmetrical tympanitic note on percussion, and the vital signs are stable, the needle is withdrawn. The small stab incision is slightly enlarged and dilated further with curved haemostat (mosquito) forceps to the size of the trocar. The incision should not be over-extended because this will cause leakage of gas. The enlarged incision should allow a tight fit around the trocar (outside diameter 7 mm). The insufflation apparatus should be attended by the circulating nurse and switched to automatic before the trocar is inserted.

The operated abdomen

Abdominal scars from previous operations do not constitute an absolute contraindication to the procedure but it is recommended that these cases should only be undertaken by the experienced laparoscopist.

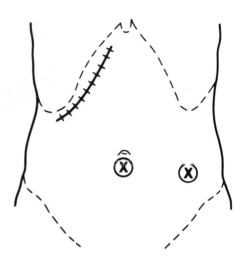

Fig 5 9 *Right subcostal incision.* The site of insertion is either in the midline below the umbilicus or in the left lower quadrant (umbilicus–iliac crest line, lateral third).

Right subcostal incision. In patients with previous cholecystectomy (subcostal incision) the site of needle puncture (Figure 5.9) can be below the umbilicus, similarly to the normal non-operated abdomen, or two-thirds of the way along a line from the umbilicus to the left anterior superior iliac spine. In general, the quadrant diametrically opposite to the site of the previous operation should be selected. The insertion of the pneumoperitoneum needle is the same as described above for the normal abdomen and the pneumoperitoneum is created and checked in a similar way. It is very important to be aware of signs indicating the presence of adhesions, for example a sudden increase in the intra-abdominal pressure or the development of an asymmetric pneumoperitoneum, diagnosed by percussion. These should be recognized early, and appropriate adjustments to the needle position should be made. Such precautions reduce the risk of perforating underlying organs, which may be bound to the abdominal wall by adhesions.

Upper midline incision. In these cases the site chosen is two-thirds of the way along a line from the umbilicus to the iliac crest in the right or left lower quadrant (Figure 5.10). The quadrant site selected is influenced by the nature of the previous operation.

Left subcostal incision. This is a mirror image of the right subcostal incision and, therefore, the right lower quadrant or sub-umbilical position should be chosen (Figure 5.11).

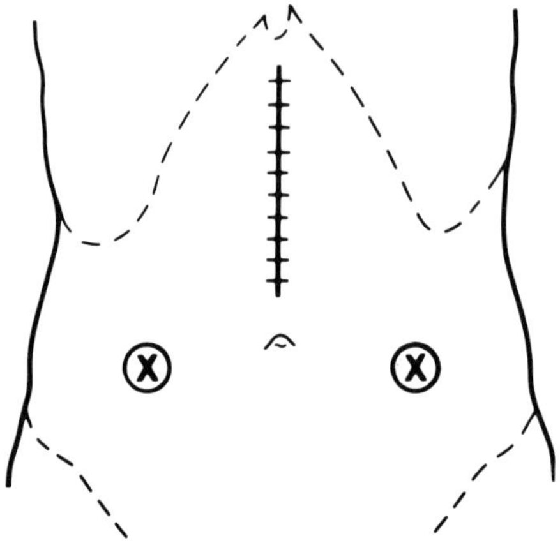

Fig. 5.10 *Upper midline incision.* Depending on the type of operation the site of insertion can be in either the left or the right lower quadrant (umbilicus–iliac crest line, lateral third).

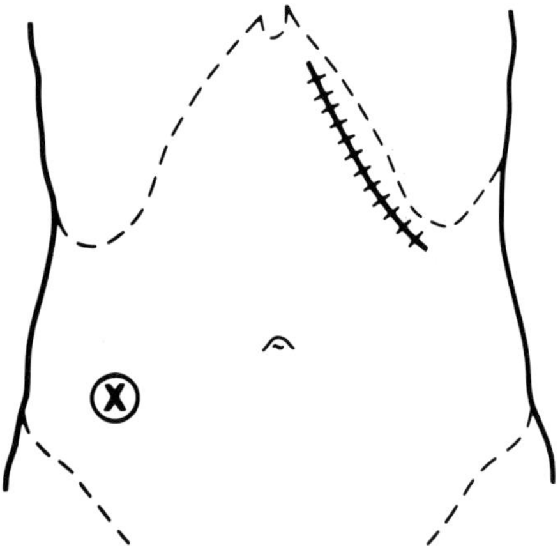

Fig. 5.11 *Left subcostal incision.* The approach of choice is in the right lower quadrant (umbilicus–iliac crest line, lateral third).

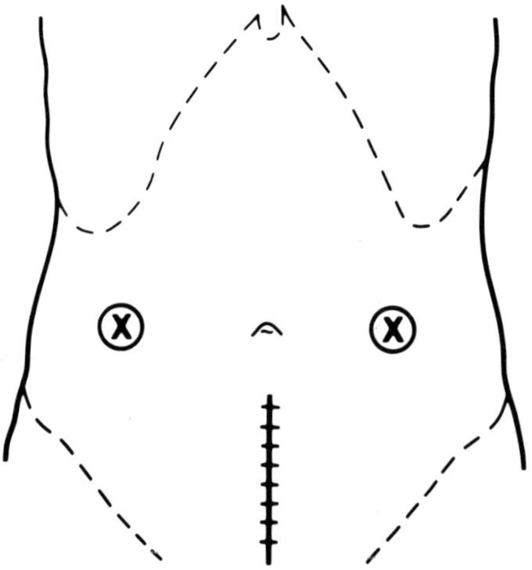

Fig. 5.12 *Lower midline incision.* Depending on the nature of the previous operation, a left or right approach at the level of the umbilicus along the linea semilunaris (the lateral edge of the rectus muscle) is used.

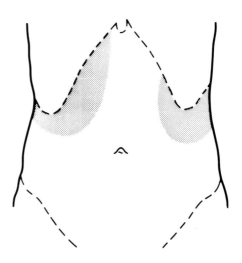

Fig. 5.13 Always examine the abdomen before a laparoscopy. In patients with a palpable liver or spleen, the surface markings of the edges of the enlarged organ(s) should be outlined with ink on the skin. This precaution avoids injuries during penetration by the Veress needle or laparoscopy trocar.

Lower midline incision. If the patient does not have hepatosplenomegaly, the site of insertion can be in the right or left upper quadrant above the umbilicus at the lateral edge of the rectus muscle (Figure 5.12).

In cirrhotic patients with obvious portal hypertension a left lower quadrant insertion of the needle should be selected in preference to a midline one, to avoid puncture of dilated para-umbilical veins. In patients with suspected hepatosplenomegaly one should examine the abdomen carefully to map out the positions of the enlarged organs (Figure 5.13).

Pitfalls

The aspiration is the first and one of the most important steps during the creation of the pneumoperitoneum in both the normal and the operated abdomen. If any blood is aspirated the needle position should be changed. If repeat aspiration is negative, insufflation and laparoscopy can commence. Care should be taken to examine the area under the needle insertion. It is not uncommon to find a large haematoma in the mesentery, mesocolon or omentum. By itself, this does not constitute an indication for exploration but close postoperative observation is important as these patients can continue bleeding or develop a transient ileus. If a vein in the mesentery is ruptured and after reposition of the needle negative aspiration is obtained, the procedure is continued and similar precautionary measures are taken as described above. If the lumen of the intestine is entered, as shown by aspiration of yellowish fluid, the needle should not be moved around because this will enlarge the hole. After repositioning and negative aspiration the procedure is continued. Thereafter a nasogastric tube should be inserted and the patient kept on intravenous fluids with close observation over the next 24–48 hours. These patients should receive systemic broad-spectrum antibiotics. Immediate laparotomy is necessary for those patients in whom trauma to any hollow viscus is more extensive than a needle puncture and whenever bowel contents are seen oozing out through the trauma site. Active bleeding seen at laparoscopy which cannot be controlled easily by electrocoagulation is also an indication for immediate surgical exploration.

If during the pneumoperitoneum or insufflation subcutaneous emphysema is created, as shown by crepitus on palpation of the abdominal wall, this indicates leakage of gas into the subcutaneous tissue around the cannula because of too large an entry hole.

In males an existing inguinal indirect hernia can result in a pneumo-scrotum. If the operator discovers the hernia in time, a truss or pressure bandage can prevent this transient phenomenon. An umbilical hernia in ascitic patients is not a contraindication.

In the operated abdomen, if the intra-abdominal pressure still exceeds the safe limit after repositioning the needle two or three times, or if there is no significant flow (indicating entanglement in massive adhesions), the following alternative can be considered. A 5 cm area around the needle insertion is infiltrated with local anaesthetic and a cutdown is made through the skin, subcutaneous tissue and muscle to the posterior sheath and peritoneum. A purse-string suture is placed in the posterior rectus sheath and then the peritoneum is opened. If there are no adhesions underneath, the trocar is inserted (without stylet) through the opening. By traction on the purse-string a tight closure around the trocar is achieved and creation of the pneumoperitoneum can be commenced. In these cases, should the intra-abdominal pressure suddenly increase within the first minute, the trocar is probably in an inflated omental sac. This can be seen if the telescope is introduced gently. This technique can also be used for a second look in operated cases where adhesions are anticipated.

When creating a pneumoperitoneum, careful observation is required to detect changes in the patient's haemodynamic, cardiac and respiratory state. During the initial learning period it is advisable not only to become acquainted with the technique of laparoscopy but also to know when to discontinue the procedure.

TROCAR INSERTION

Standard trocar

When the pneumoperitoneum is completed, the needle is withdrawn. The stab incision is enlarged with the blade slightly and stretched with a haemostat forceps just sufficiently to accept a standard 7mm trocar (Figure 5.14). The skin incision should not be deep because gas leakage can occur. The trocar is held in one hand in a fist, employing a drilling–pressing action after the sharp stylet is

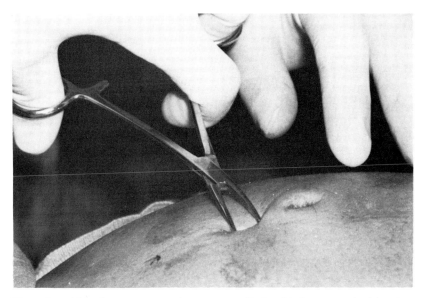

Fig. 5.14   After the pneumoperitoneum needle is withdrawn, an incision is made in the skin only. It is then stretched with a haemostat forceps to accommodate the trocar. The incision should be a tight fit; otherwise gas will escape beside the trocar.

inserted into the opening of the skin. The index finger and thumb of the other hand hold the trocar sleeve, as a 'brake' (Figure 5.15). As soon as resistance is lost, this 'brake' prevents further advancement of the trocar and prevents injury to internal organs. (Alternatively, the instrument is held with the index finger along the trocar shaft with the end of the finger one inch (2.5cm) away from the tip of the trocar, such that the finger acts as a brake when the peritoneum is punctured.) Then the pressing–drilling hand is removed. A hissing noise indicates that the trocar tip is correctly positioned in the peritoneum. The stylet is withdrawn and the trocar sleeve advanced

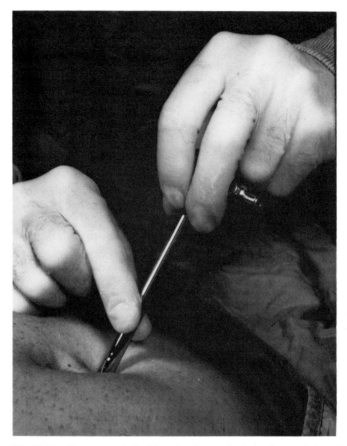

Fig. 5.15   The trocar is held in the fist with the index and thumb of the other hand holding the trocar as a 'brake'. It is advanced with a drilling–pressing action. If the procedure is performed under local anaesthesia, the patient is instructed to lift up his or her head to tighten the abdominal muscles. As soon as resistance is lost, further advancement of the trocar is stopped. A hissing noise should be heard, indicating that the inflated peritoneal cavity has been entered.

about one inch (2.5 cm), roughly parallel to the abdominal wall. In obese abdominal walls it is very important to create a tight pneumoperitoneum to facilitate safe penetration. When the procedure is performed under local anaesthesia, the patient is asked to lift up his or her head and keep it up for a few seconds during the penetration as the resulting contraction of the abdominal muscles during the manoeuvre increases the resistance to the advancing trocar and facilitates safe insertion.

If several unsuccessful attempts have been made, the procedure should be abandoned because the trocar may perforate vital organs. In ascitic patients or cachectic patients an extremely thin abdominal wall can be easily and suddenly penetrated so less drilling pressure is advisable.

Accessory trocar

The second, accessory trocar and cannula should be introduced whenever feasible, to palpate and lift organs, obtain fluid or tissue samples, etc. The probe is the extension of the operator's finger. The site chosen for insertion is dependent on the location of pathology and can be further assessed by viewing through the telescope while indenting the abdominal wall with the index finger (Figure 5.16). This will confirm if the selected site for insertion of accessory trocar is optimal in relation to the pathology and free of underlying adhesions

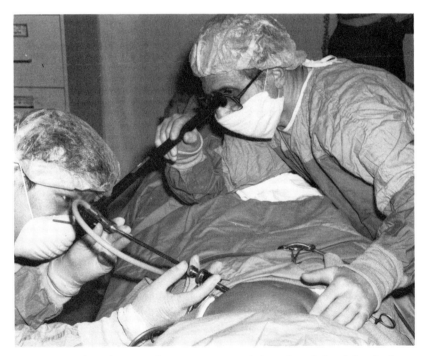

Fig. 5.16   Before the second accessory trocar is introduced the abdominal wall is indented by a finger and the resulting localized protrusion of the peritoneal lining is visualized. In this way the optimal site for the insertion of the second trocar can be selected. The transillumination of the abdominal wall also facilitates the identification of dilated veins, if present.

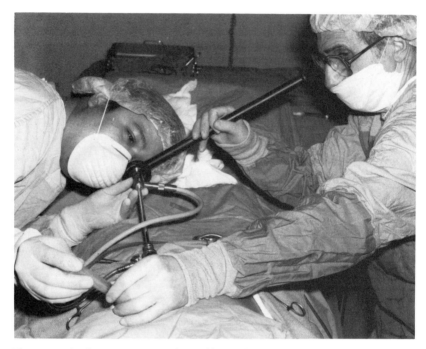

Fig. 5.17   1% lignocaine is used to infiltrate the selected site. The penetration of the needle is observed through the telescope.

or loops of bowel. During the insertion of the accessory trocar it is very important to avoid injuries to the epigastric vessels. The site of insertion should therefore be along the lateral edge of the rectus (linea semilunaris). If the procedure is being performed under local anaesthesia, the selected site is infiltrated as previously described (Figure 5.17). A small stab incision is made through the skin only. This is slightly enlarged with a curved haemostat (mosquito) forceps, just enough to accept a 4mm trocar sleeve. The accessory trocar with its stylet is held in one hand and penetration of the abdominal wall is achieved by a drilling–pressing action while the other hand holds the telescope (Figure 5.18). The protruding tip of the stylet is thus kept under vision and can be directed with safety. Because of the confined space between the parietal peritoneum and underlying organs the sharp tip is aimed in an oblique fashion *towards the telescope*, so avoiding injuries to the underlying organs. As soon as the trocar has penetrated the parietal peritoneum, the stylet is withdrawn and the valve closed. The palpation probe is advanced through the trocar sleeve after the valve is opened and a systematic examination is begun (Figures 5.18–5.20).

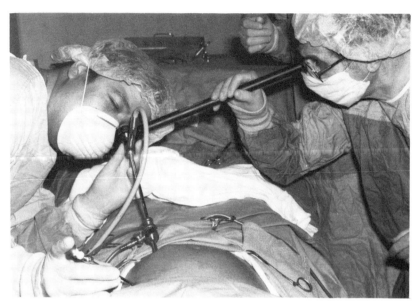

Fig. 5.18 After a skin incision is made the second trocar is inserted under visual control. The trocar is guided towards the telescope in order to avoid injury to the underlying organs.

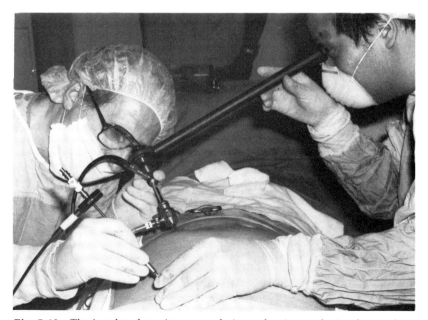

Fig. 5.19 The insulated suction–coagulation palpation probe is advanced and its appearance observed through a telescope.

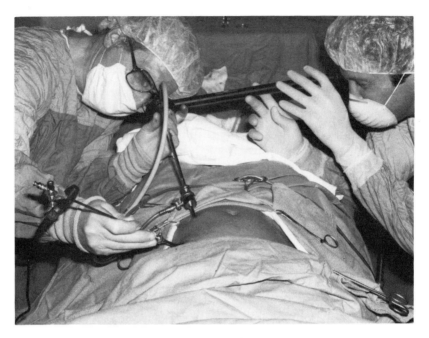

Fig. 5.20   The palpation probe is essential for good laparoscopic inspection; it is the workhorse of laparoscopy and acts as an extension of the operator's finger. Organs can be palpated and lifted, and one should never perform a biopsy without palpating the organ beforehand.

When the pathology is on the anterior surface of the parietal peritoneum above the right lobe of the liver, right diaphragm or in the supracolic compartment, the optimal approach is beneath the right costal margin and along the lateral edge of the rectus muscle. Even a lesion in the left lobe of the liver can be approached carefully from the right side by advancing the probe or forceps under the ligamentum teres.

If the initial approach is unsuccessful or the pathology cannot be reached and the accessory trocar is already inserted, a third small trocar should be introduced without hesitation or the second trocar should be repositioned in a site suitable for obtaining tissue samples with safety. The small stab incisions, which are closed with skin clips, are hardly visible after a few months.

Large trocar

A larger trocar (O.D. 11 mm) is required for photography and television because the telescope contains more fibres. Therefore, a slightly larger incision is needed. It is very important to introduce this trocar *with great care* and with the same technique as described above in order to avoid injuries to the underlying organs.

INSERTION OF THE TELESCOPE

The telescope has to be pre-warmed. There are various ways to do this. We use a sterile container which is filled with warm saline in which the telescope is immersed. After the trocar is in position the telescope is removed from the container and is dried before it is inserted into the trocar sheath. The fibre-optic cable is connected. The observation is begun when the telescope is in the sheath. Do not 'poke' the telescope into the abdominal cavity without simultaneous observation (Figure 5.21).

You should see the distal hole of the metal tunnel within the sheath and be able to recognize the entry into the abdominal cavity immediately. As the telescope is forward-oblique looking, during introduction the direction of view should be aimed towards the

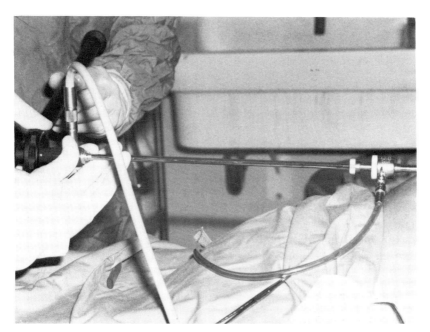

Fig. 5.21 Do not insert the telescope blindly into the cannula. As soon as it is introduced, observe further advancement and make sure that you can see the exit from this metal sheath into the cavity.

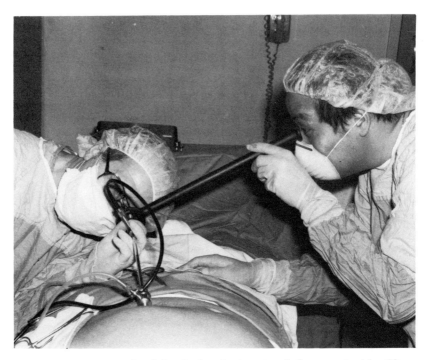

Fig. 5.22   As soon as the abdominal cavity is entered, the operator identifies the landmarks: the ligamentum teres (round ligament) and falciform ligament.

intra-abdominal organs or retroperitoneum. This is easy to check if you observe the connection of the fibre-optic cable. If this is positioned upwards (towards the ceiling) the working end of the optic looks downwards. On entering the abdomen, the first landmark in the upper abdomen which you should look for is the round ligament (teres) and its attached falciform ligament (Figure 5.22). If the telescope end is smudged with a few drops of blood, the view will become foggy. In this case the telescope is withdrawn and immersed in warm saline and wiped. Do not remove blood or fluid from the tip of the telescope by wiping with a dry gauze because this will only further interfere with good vision. Always ensure that the optic is crystal-clear.

DESUFFLATION

At the conclusion of the examination the telescope is withdrawn. The trocar valve is kept open to desufflate the abdomen. Gentle pressure can be exerted on the abdominal wall while the trocar is slowly withdrawn. Too rapid a removal of the trocar can cause omentum to be dragged into the wound. Should this happen, it can be replaced in the peritoneal cavity with dissecting forceps. The skin incision can be closed with skin clips or interrupted mattress sutures.

6

Inspection of the Abdominal Cavity

ORIENTATION

Inspection should start as soon as the pre-warmed and dried telescope is introduced into the trocar. The operator turns the forward-oblique telescope to view downwards (towards abdominal organs) and holds it in this position. Initially the tubular appearance of the inside of the trocar is seen. The trocar should be held *parallel* to the abdomen wall as this avoids entangling the advancing tip of the telescope in the omentum. If yellowish tissue is seen immediately in front of the trocar sleeve the telescope is either in the pre-peritoneal fat or among dense adhesions. When the free abdominal cavity has been clearly recognized, inspection starts with the recognition of the first landmark – the falciform ligament. The liver is inspected next. It is useful to keep the telescope two to three inches (5–8 cm) from the liver to obtain a good overview. If some displacement of organ is discovered, this can indicate possible sources of pathology. Next the telescope is turned 180° to inspect the diaphragmatic and parietal peritoneum. The normal appearance of this is a smooth shiny pink membrane with a delicate vascular network. Abnormalities include dilated vessels indicative of portal hypertension, hyperaemia and inflammation, adhesions and discrete flat ulcerated or elevated lesions, which can be localized or widespread. Sometimes the diaphragm is obliterated from vision by dense adhesions.

The next step is to ascertain if there is fluid in the paracolic gutters. If so, is it straw coloured or haemorrhagic? Is it chylous or turbulent? Is the undersurface of the liver visible at all?

Can the gallbladder be recognized, and, if so, is it distended or normal in appearance? Moving the telescope carefully under the round ligament towards the left upper quadrant, the left lobe should be visualized. Under normal conditions the spleen is not visible because it is covered with omentum. The inspection of the parietal peritoneum from this position is performed in the same way as on the right side. Observing the left lobe of the liver, is it normal in size? Is it small or enlarged (which is common in cirrhosis)? If the lobes of the liver are covered by omentum, the patient can be tilted in a reversed Trendelenburg position. This can help to move the omentum spontaneously. If not, using a palpation probe introduced through a second trocar, one can gently move the omentum away from the liver. Force should not be used with this manoeuvre if resistance due to adhesions is encountered.

The anterior surface of the stomach can be seen behind and below the lobe of the liver. In cases of portal hypertension the dilated veins on the omentum and on the greater curvature of the stomach are well displayed. If the lower pole or anterior edge of the spleen is visible this indicates possible splenomegaly. If the spleen requires inspection it is best to rotate the patient to the right and increase the reversed Trendelenburg position. Below the greater curvature of the stomach the splenic flexure of the colon with taeniae can be recognized.

In the presence of ascitic fluid, the parietal peritoneum can be hyperaemic, inflamed, or dull in appearance. To inspect the pelvic area, the telescope is pulled back into the trocar sheath, the patient is placed in the horizontal position, the trocar is turned counterclockwise to the pelvic area and the telescope is then advanced for inspection of the lower abdomen. In patients with suspected pelvic pathology or gynaecological disorders, a previously inserted Foley catheter can be used to identify the bladder; this can be helpful in avoiding bladder trauma if the accessory trocar has to be introduced above the symphysis pubis. At this stage the Trendelenburg position greatly improves the view.

INSPECTION OF THE ABDOMINAL ORGANS

The first landmark should be the round ligament (ligamentum teres) and the falciform ligament. The ligamentum teres is a fibro-adipose cord, representing the obliterated umbilical vein, which extends from above the umbilicus towards the porta hepatis and is attached to the left branch of the portal vein. It has a fatty appearance with fine vessels. Its continuation above the liver lobes is formed by the falciform ligament, which is also attached to the diaphragm. The falciform ligament is sickle-shaped, opaque and sometimes infiltrated with fat and contains a few fine vessels. It forms a curtain-like partition above the anterior surface of the liver and can be observed from both sides.

Liver lobes

The normal liver is reddish-brown with a smooth, shiny surface. The edges are sharp towards the lateral aspects of both lobes. The medial aspect of each lobe dips towards the falciform ligament. The capsule may be smooth or thickened.

Subcapsular fibrosis produces a whitish appearance and thickening of the capsule and can be circumscribed or diffuse. Fibrosis of Glisson's capsule can follow surgical intervention, peritonitis or ascites. Very thin, curtain-like adhesions between the parietal peritoneum and the anterior surface of the liver lobes can cause severe symptoms such as right upper quadrant pain. If laparoscopy is performed under local anaesthesia the pain can be provoked by gentle pressure with the palpation probe on the liver lobe or on the adhesions. This peri-hepatitis can be of inflammatory origin (Fitz-Hugh–Curtis syndrome). Occasionally, small (1–2mm) whitish, soft nodules can be found in this condition. These may consist of condensations of mesothelial collagen tissue or lymph collections. Metastatic lesions are solid and hard.

The appearance of the left lobe should be similar to that of the right. Under normal conditions the inferior surface of the liver is not visible. In cases of hypertrophy, fibrosis, infiltration by metastases or retroperitoneal mass, the inferior surface is more readily seen.

Gallbladder

The normal gallbladder in a fasting patient is slightly distended, and the peritoneal surface is *shiny* greenish-blue in colour as the thin-walled gallbladder transmits the colour of the bile. Small tortuous blood vessels are seen on the surface. The pathological gallbladder appears pale, whitish or opaque. For better inspection a palpating probe should be introduced. The lateral edge of the right lobe can be gently lifted with the palpating probe positioned beneath it. With this manoeuvre the gallbladder is more easily inspected. Omental adhesions to the gallbladder indicate chronic or past inflammation (cholecystitis).

Stomach

In most cases the anterior wall, including parts of the duodenum, antrum and body can be seen below the liver. The greater curvature with the gastro-epiploic arcade can be observed. If the stomach is significantly distended, this can interfere with the examination of the liver lobes, so aspiration via a nasogastric tube is recommended.

Spleen

The normal spleen is not visible with the patient in the supine position since it is covered with omentum. If splenic visualization is necessary, rotation of the patient to the right and the steep reversed Trendelenburg position is required. The omentum can be very gently teased down with the palpation probe, but careful attention has to be paid to the spleno-colic ligament: over-stretching this can result in tearing of the splenic capsule, with severe bleeding. The spleen appears bluish-brown in colour. There may be a few notches seen on the medial margin; these are much more pronounced in splenomegaly.

Omentum

The appearance and the extent of the omentum correlates with the patient's build and specifically the weight. The thin or cachectic patient has insignificant, filmy omentum whereas in an obese patient this fatty apron can be extremely thick, covering most of the intra-abdominal organs, and be difficult to move with the palpating probe. In some instances it can obscure the right or left lobe of the liver, but with careful manipulation it can be moved. This can be facilitated by placing the patient in a reversed Trendelenburg position. The omental veins are grossly dilated in portal hypertension, often reaching a diameter of 4–5 mm. In this situation, great care is needed when manipulating the omentum as rupture of one of these veins can result in severe bleeding.

Peritoneum

By rotating the telescope within its sheath through 180°, away from the intra-abdominal organs, the parietal peritoneum can be inspected. Under normal conditions the peritoneum is pinkish-white in colour and has a fine vascular architecture. Dilated peritoneal vessels suggest the presence of portal hypertension. These dilated vessels are particularly evident in the diaphragmatic peritoneum above the liver. It is usual in this area to see an artery in between two adjacent veins.

In the right upper quadrant an indentation of the peritoneum covering the dome of the right lobe can be encountered. This is called the Zahn's indentation and can simulate a filling defect on isotope or CT scans. As the peritoneal lining over the diaphragm is very thin, the muscular and the tendinous sections of the diaphragm can be well distinguished. On the left side (left upper quadrant) the pulsation of the heart can be seen through this structure. Diaphragmatic metastases (ovarian carcinomas) appear as small whitish nodules. It is advisable to biopsy these lesions very carefully with a punch forceps to avoid perforation.

After the upper abdominal (parietal) surface is observed, the telescope can be withdrawn into the trocar sheath under visual control and the telescope, with the trocar, turned towards the pelvic area. The telescope is advanced and the appearance of the parietal peritoneum in the lower quadrants of the abdomen and pelvis observed. In females or in patients with suspected pelvic pathology, the second (accessory) trocar is often introduced above the symphysis. A previously inserted Foley catheter provides a good landmark of the intraperitoneal part of the bladder and will help to avoid inadvertent perforation of this organ.

Pancreas and small bowel

These require special manoeuvres and are considered in Chapter 9.

Female pelvic organs

Gynaecological laparoscopy is dealt with in Chapter 12.

INSPECTION IN SPECIFIC DISORDERS

Cirrhotic liver

The appearance of the liver architecture helps to confirm progressive cirrhosis. An irregular surface, nodularity, or fibrosis with regenerating nodules of varying sizes are common. The cirrhotic liver is indurated and stiff when palpated, and the inferior surface, which under normal conditions is not seen, is projected into the visual field. In certain instances the cirrhotic liver is pale, but this appearance can change, with reddish discolouration between the normal and regenerating liver parenchyma. Small tortuous vessels are visible on the surface, especially if the process is in the active phase, but can be associated also with portal hypertension. Small white, soft-appearing nodules on the anterior surface can represent lymphatic blebs. In the end-stage the liver is small, shrunken, hard and contains large nodules. These nodules are demarcated by deep bands of fibrous tissue.

The appearance of the liver alone often provides the diagnostic clue. Nodules over 3mm are indicative of macronodular cirrhosis; in contrast micronodular cirrhosis is characterized by smaller nodules which are diffuse and irregular in appearance, resulting in a coarse granular surface. This distinction is rather artificial and there are many cirrhotic livers where the appearance is mixed, consisting of both large and small nodules.

Fatty degeneration appears as a yellowish, mottled change on the liver surface, with or without micronodular changes. This is very often found in patients with alcohol abuse. Larger macronodular nodules with a bluish tint on the surface may indicate the presence of a post-necrotic cirrhosis especially in the younger patient.

Cholestasis

We have reported the advantages of laparoscopic percutaneous transhepatic cholecystocholangiography in the differentiation between extra-hepatic biliary obstruction due to stones, or neoplasm and hepatocellular jaundice.[1,2,3] The procedure displays the extra- and intrahepatic bile ducts with great precision. However, the development of diagnostic ultrasound, the introduction of fine-needle percutaneous transhepatic cholangiography and the availability of endoscopic retrograde cholangiography have largely replaced laparoscopy in the differentiation and/or diagnosis of the patient with problematic cholestasis.

If laparoscopy is performed for other reasons and a distended gallbladder is found which on palpation or slight compression remains tense and the liver is greenish or dark green in colour, this would indicate an extrahepatic obstruction, probably due to pancreatic or periampullary cancer. The degree of greenish colouration of the liver does not correlate with the serum bilirubin level. The collapsed gallbladder suggests an intrahepatic cholestasis, e.g., drug-induced jaundice or tumour at the hilar bifurcation (Klatskin tumour).

In patients with advanced cirrhosis, the gallbladder is often observed to be enlarged at laparoscopy. However, it can be easily compressed with the palpation probe, indicating that there is no distal obstruction. The aetiology of this distended gallbladder is not known. A collapsed gallbladder, with a normal appearance, excludes distal common bile duct obstruction. If a liver biopsy is contemplated in a patient with a suspected hepato-cellular disease and a tissue core is obtained, it is advisable to compress or coagulate the area to ensure that no bile leakage occurs and to minimize the risk of bleeding.

Portal hypertension

Laparoscopy provides an excellent assessment of an intrahepatic block causing portal hypertension, and demonstrates the characteristic appearance of dilated veins on the parietal peritoneum, ligamentum teres or omentum, together with evidence of splenomegaly.

Metastatic liver lesions

At present there is no other test available including isotope, ultrasound or CT scan, liver function tests etc., which has the high sensitivity and specificity of a target liver biopsy under visual control. In 90% of patients with metastatic liver disease, lesions are visible on the liver surface as isolated yellowish–whitish nodules just below the capsule, multiple nodules or diffuse infiltration of the parenchyma. Sometimes the deposits form round, circumscribed firm nodules, elevated slightly, but with a central crater resulting from necrosis (umbilicated). The edges can be hypervascular, with small telan-giectatic vessels surrounding these lesions. They can sometimes be so extensive in number that only a few areas of normal liver surface are visible amongst the infiltrating metastatic lesions.

In metastatic malignant melanoma, the deposits appear as round, dark brown or black spots just slightly protruding or flush with the liver surface.

Carcinoid tumours also can produce whitish, circumscribed nodules, or large intraparenchymal lesions protruding towards the surface and are easily seen in a tangential view.

Rarely, a metastatic lesion is located only intra-parenchymally but it can be recognized from the bulging liver surface. With the palpation probe, the suspected areas feel harder than the surrounding normal liver parenchyma.

Primary carcinoma of the liver

This can be small, nodular in appearance and involve one or both lobes. These tumours have a good blood supply and therefore necrosis with the crater-like formation is not often encountered. Sometimes a small primary lesion can cause diffuse widespread nodules on the parietal peritoneum. Hepatocellular carcinoma occurs more frequently in a cirrhotic liver. It is important to think of this entity in a cirrhotic patient if the clinical picture suddenly deteriorates. Very careful inspection and systematic palpation is necessary and must include the undersurface of the liver (see also Chapter 8).

Lymphoma

In Hodgkin's disease the presence of splenomegaly and nodules on the anterior surface of the liver as well as on the visible part of the spleen can confirm the metastatic stage of this disease. The infiltrated liver in Hodgkin's disease is enlarged and on palpation gives the impression of a 'stiff' organ. The pattern of the liver parenchyma is disrupted and small patches or nodules of various sizes elevated beyond the liver surface are observed. A Hodgkin's lymphoma can occur as a circumscribed area where the parenchyma has been replaced by numerous soft whitish irregular lesions or it can appear as diffuse nodular soft yellowish–whitish lesions with irregular star-shaped but well defined margins disseminated on both lobes. Large numbers of minute whitish spots which distort the known pattern of the liver surface can also be present.

The laparoscopic inspection of the spleen in Hodgkin's disease with intraparenchymal lesions is less effective than surgical exploration at splenectomy. In non-Hodgkin's lymphomas the extrahepatic metastases can be discovered with ease and tissue samples obtained.

Benign tumours

Hamartomas and adenomas are rare. They are usually localized in one lobe. Haemangiomas are more common. They appear as bluish lesions which on palpation have a cystic consistency. Laparoscopic biopsy is positively contraindicated in these and all fluid-filled hepatic lesions. Haemangiomas are also characterized by a smooth surface, but with coarse fibrous trabeculae which give an impression of partitions, but if palpated a soft consistency will be ascertained.

REFERENCES

1   Berci, G., Morgenstern, L., Shore, J.M. & Shapiro, S. (1973) A direct approach to the differential diagnosis of jaundice. Laparoscopy with transhepatic cholecystocholangiography. *Am. J. Surg.* 126: 372–378.
2   Cuschieri, A. (1975) Value of laparoscopy in hepatobiliary disease. *Ann. R. Coll. Surg. Eng.* 57: 33–38.
3   Irving, A.D. & Cuschieri, A. (1978) Laparoscopic assessment of the jaundiced patient. *Br. J. Surg.* 65: 678–680.

7

Tissue Sampling Techniques

One of the main advantages of laparoscopy is the ability to obtain guided biopsies or tissue for cytological examination which allows the establishment of a definitive diagnosis. However, certain precautions are necessary to ensure the complete safety of these procedures and preoperative evaluation of the blood clotting mechanism is essential.

PREOPERATIVE EVALUATION

In the first instance a history of any bleeding tendency must be obtained in addition to details of drug therapy. The haemoglobin level, prothrombin time, kaolin-cephalin time and platelet count are measured. Jaundiced patients with an elevated prothrombin time are treated with intramuscular vitamin K analogue and the prothrombin time then repeated 24–36 hours later. This therapy should reduce the prolonged prothrombin time if this is the result of malabsorption of vitamin K consequent on the obstructive jaundice. Hepatocellular decompensation is diagnosed if the prolonged prothrombin time is unaltered by vitamin K therapy. If such a patient requires a laparoscopic biopsy, the entire procedure should be covered with fresh frozen plasma, started preoperatively. Platelet transfusions are administered before the procedure to patients whose platelet count is below 50×10^9/l. If the thrombocytopenia is less severe, platelet units should be available in case of bleeding following the biopsy but preoperative platelet transfusion is unnecessary.

BIOPSY INSTRUMENTS

These include sharp-pointed and punch biopsy forceps, needle core biopsy sets (Tru-cut, long-shaft Menghini and Vim-Silverman) a fine needle aspiration cytology set (Chiba gauge 23), brush cytology equipment and the laparoscopic suction cannula for peritoneal washings.

INITIAL LAPAROSCOPIC ASSESSMENT

The procedure should always commence with a thorough laparoscopic inspection of the peritoneal cavity and its contents aided by the use of the palpating probe introduced through the accessory trocar. The pathology is thus defined and the optimum site for insertion of biopsy equipment (irrespective of type used) is determined by the finger compression technique (Chapter 5). In addition *it is essential that the lesion is palpated before a biopsy is taken* to differentiate between a solid and a cystic lesion. Forceps and needle core biopsies are contraindicated in all cystic lesions within the peritoneal cavity but there is no objection to aspiration via a fine Chiba needle. Manifestly vascular lesions, particularly haemangioma of the liver, should never be biopsied by any technique. The use of the rigid teaching attachment greatly assists all laparoscopic biopsy procedures as it allows both surgeon and assistant complete visual control throughout the entire procedure.

FORCEPS BIOPSY

This is the best biopsy technique for *exophytic lesions* on the surface of the liver and intestines and for biopsy of the parietal peritoneum including that lining the undersurface of the diaphragm. Forceps biopsy is the best method of establishing a definitive diagnosis in tuberculous peritonitis and for primary and secondary tumours of the parietal peritoneum.

The biopsy forceps is introduced via an accessory cannula at a site appropriate to the location of the lesion to be biopsied (Figure 7.1). A 45° angle between the line of the trocar penetration and the intended biopsy is the best approach. Once the forceps is seen within the peritoneal cavity, its jaws are opened and closed to determine the direction of jaw movement in relation to the lesion. With the instrument held in the open position the fixed jaw, which is a continuation of the stem of the biopsy forceps, is inserted just beside the lesion (Figure 7.2). During expiration, the mobile jaw of the forceps is then closed, the instrument withdrawn and the tissue sample recovered. The specimen is then carefully removed from the jaws of the instrument by means of a hypodermic needle and placed on a piece of sterile cardboard. It is then handed to the nurse to be placed in formaldehyde solution. Some tissue samples may need to be cultured (e.g., suspected tuberculosis), in which case part of the sample is placed in a sterile container and sent immediately to the bacteriology laboratory. Other samples, particularly some liver biopsies, may need examination by electron microscopy and thus require fixation in gluteraldehyde solution.

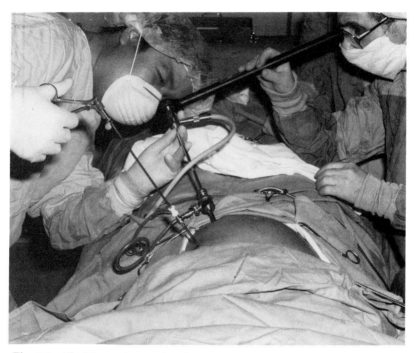

Fig. 7.1   The biopsy forceps is advanced through the accessory cannula under visual control. Assistants may observe the procedure through the teaching attachment.

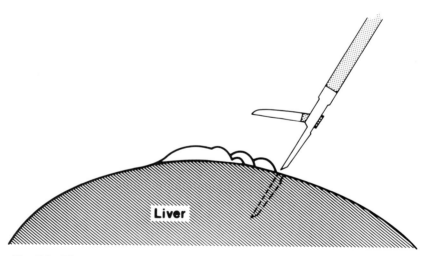

Fig. 7.2   The pointed tip forceps is used for exophytic surface liver lesions. Its fixed jaw is inserted beside the lesion. The upper mobile jaw is then closed to obtain a tissue sample.

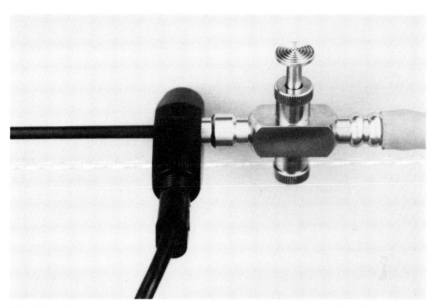

Fig. 7.3   The insulated suction–coagulation–palpating probe should always be available. It is connected to the suction machine and via a high-frequency cable to an electrosurgical unit for coagulation.

The biopsy site is then inspected by the viewing telescope. The previously inserted suction–coagulation–palpating probe is connected both to the suction machine and to the electrosurgical unit (Figure 7.3) and the patient's contact with the plate from the electrosurgical unit is checked. The biopsy site is then coagulated if bleeding continues despite direct local pressure with the palpating probe. The same procedure is repeated if more than one biopsy is considered necessary. Some of the peritoneal CO_2 is lost during these manipulations so the pneumoperitoneum cushion has to be maintained by further insufflation.

The pointed tip biopsy forceps is ideal for biopsy of exophytic hepatic lesions. In other locations, however, e.g. diaphragm, parietal peritoneum and the intestinal surface, the punch forceps is preferable and safer since it cuts a portion of tissue within its cups without the risk of tearing the underlying organ (Figures 7.4 and 7.5).

CORE NEEDLE BIOPSY

This technique is used for the biopsy of flat hepatic lesions, diffuse cirrhosis of the liver and large intra-abdominal masses. Both the Tru-cut and long-shaft Menghini needles obtain a deep core biopsy.

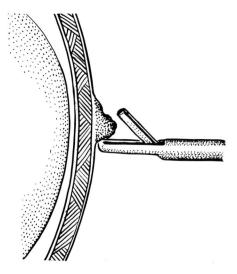

Fig. 7.4   In lesions on the diaphragm and parietal peritoneum and on the surface of the intestines, the punch forceps is employed to avoid tearing or injuries to the underlying organ.

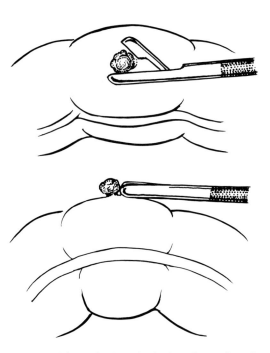

Fig. 7.5   The technique for lesions located on the serosa of the intestine. The punch forceps has sharp cup-shaped edges which cut cleanly without tearing the adjacent tissues and underlying organ.

In practice there is little to choose between these two needles despite claims to the contrary, and one should become familiar with the use of one or the other. The Vim-Silverman needle is inferior to both the Tru-cut and the Menghini and is rarely used nowadays.

Tru-cut biopsy

Having ascertained the appropriate site of insertion, a small stab incision is made in the skin with a fine-pointed scalpel and the Tru-cut needle inserted through the abdominal wall in the closed position. The needle is then guided under visual control towards the intended site of the biopsy (Figure 7.6). With the patient in expiration, and the needle in the open position, its sharp stylet is advanced into the lesion or liver substance. The outer cutting sheath is then pushed down until it goes no further. In so doing it cuts a core of tissue. The closed needle is withdrawn. While the assistant is removing the tissue sample from the needle, the operator compresses the biopsy site with the palpating probe. If bleeding continues thereafter, electrocautery is applied to the puncture site.

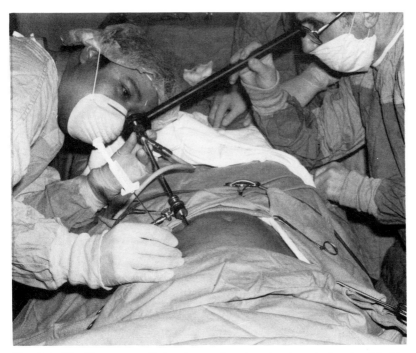

Fig. 7.6   The Tru-cut needle is advanced under visual control and guided to the intended biopsy site.

Menghini biopsy

The Menghini needle/stylet assembly is introduced in the same way as the Tru-cut needle. Then the stylet is removed and the nail (blocking pin) is introduced into the needle shaft. Next, the Menghini needle is attached to a 20 ml syringe containing 10 ml saline and its tip is guided to the intended biopsy site under telescopic vision. At this stage a few millilitres of saline are injected to clear the needle of any accumulated tissue fragments. With the patient in apnoea in the expiratory phase the needle is inserted into the lesion or liver and withdrawn in one movement while suction is applied by the assistant. The nail inside the lumen of the needle shaft ensures that the core of tissue obtained remains in the needle and is not fragmented and sucked into the syringe barrel. The specimen is retrieved by ejection of saline, which forces the tissue sample out on to a piece of sterile cardboard placed on top of a sterile gauze swab.

CYTOLOGY

Cellular material can be obtained during laparoscopy in three ways: by brush cytology, from peritoneal washings and by fine needle aspiration.

Brush cytology

This is used alone or in combination with biopsy. In our experience the best technique is to introduce the brush within its outer plastic sheath through the suction cannula, since this allows better guidance by imparting rigidity to the assembly. The trumpet valve has to be kept open by the operator continually to allow the advancement or placement of the sheathed brush. A rubber 'nipple plug' with a small hole has to be placed on the probe to avoid loss of pneumoperi-toneum. The brush, with its outer plastic sheath, protrudes for 2.0 cm beyond the end of the cannula. The cannula is then guided to the intended site under visual control. The outer plastic sheath is retracted and brushings are taken. Next, the brush is retracted into the plastic sheath and then withdrawn through the suction cannula (Figure 7.7). Smears are made on glass slides. In addition, the brush is rinsed in polyethylene glycol cell fixative (Carbowax, Breox). The fixative is later centrifuged and cytological examination of the sediment is performed in addition to examination of the glass smear preparations.

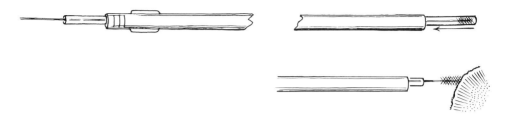

Fig. 7.7   Top: Suction cannula/brush cytology assembly. The brush within its outer sheath protrudes some 2.0 cm beyond the tip of the cannula. Bottom: the sheath has been withdrawn to expose the brush prior to obtaining brushings of the lesion.

Peritoneal washings

This technique is used in gynaecology, largely for the staging of ovarian cancer. 200–300 ml saline are injected into the pelvic cavity and then aspirated via the suction cannula. The procedure is then repeated in the subphrenic region.

Fine needle aspiration cytology

This very safe and reliable technique is especially useful for aspiration of pancreatic lesions and lymph node masses. The details of the procedure are described in Chapter 9.

Bile cytology

Cytological examination of bile aspirated from the gallbladder usually confirms the diagnosis of cancer of this organ and can also be positive in patients with pancreatic cancer. Aspiration of the gallbladder is best performed via the edge of the right lobe through the gallbladder bed using a fine Chiba needle, as outlined in Chapter 9, though some use direct puncture of the gallbladder. The latter technique may, however, lead to bile leakage into the peritoneal cavity.

8

Laparoscopy for Hepatobiliary Disease and Ascites

The reported experience on the use of laparoscopy in hepatobiliary disease is extensive and testifies to the extreme usefulness of this procedure in the diagnosis and management of patients with these disorders. No other investigative modality yields as much information relating to gross appearance, extent of the disease and degree of advancement as laparoscopy. Often the macroscopic features are in themselves diagnostic. In addition the procedure allows safe and reliable target biopsy or cytology of lesions encountered.

This chapter deals with the laparoscopic appearances of common disorders of the hepatobiliary system. In the first instance, however, beginners must familiarize themselves with the normal state of the liver, spleen and gallbladder as seen through the laparoscope. As there are many excellent colour atlases of laparoscopy, photographs of the commonly encountered conditions have not been included. None the less, a good idea of the diagnostic scope of this endoscopic procedure can be obtained by reference to the colour plates in this book. This chapter stresses the important laparoscopic changes which can be observed and which are characteristic of common specific hepatobiliary disorders.

GALLBLADDER

The gallbladder is readily visible at laparoscopy. A good examination of the organ requires concomitant use of the palpating probe to lift the edge of the right lobe of the liver and to palpate and indent the gallbladder. Other special techniques which can be useful include bile aspiration for biochemical analysis, culture and cytology and ultrasound examination.[1-5] The latter entails the use of an ultrasonic probe introduced through a second accessory cannula with scanning in the A or B mode (real time).[4-7]

Normal appearance

The normal gallbladder has a bluish glistening appearance with a smooth serosal coat containing delicate blood vessels. After elevation of the edge of the right hepatic lobe the fundus, sides and inferior surface are readily visible. The normal organ feels soft to the palpating probe and is readily compressible. Not infrequently the omentum may cover the gallbladder but is easily displaced by the palpating probe or by positional change (reversed Trendelenburg). In chronic liver disease the gallbladder, though not inflamed, is enlarged and uplifted (Plates 3 and 4). Even so it can be readily indented by the palpating probe and does not feel tense. The exact cause for this enlargement of the gallbladder in cirrhosis is not known but the current hypothesis concerns defective gallbladder emptying. *The normal gallbladder always appears full of bile at laparoscopy.*

Congenital anomalies

The most common anomalies encountered at laparoscopy include the partially intrahepatic gallbladder and the *phrygian cap*, where the fundus is constricted and turned back on itself. The fully intrahepatic gallbladder is rare. The so-called floating gallbladder, which has a complete serosal covering and a dorsal mesentery, is relatively uncommon, as is transposition of the gallbladder, either between the two hepatic lobes in the midline or underneath the left lobe. An elongated sausage-shaped gallbladder frequently accompanies congenital cystic disease of the bile duct. Another rare anomaly is the trabeculated gallbladder, but this usually causes symptoms similar to chronic cholecystitis and is associated with abnormal gallbladder emptying and dyskinesia.

Collapse/distension

As previously mentioned, the normal gallbladder appears full of bile, which contributes to its bluish appearance.

A collapsed pale gallbladder in a jaundiced patient is indicative of a cholangiocarcinoma either of the common hepatic duct or at the junction of the right and left hepatic ducts (hilar or Klatskin tumour). In this situation full elevation of the edge of the right lobe by the palpating probe may reveal the bulge caused by the tumour and any extension to the adjacent hepatic parenchyma.

An enlarged tense distended gallbladder, which does not indent on pressure with the palpating probe, indicates distal bile duct obstruction, usually from a peri-ampullary or pancreatic carcinoma. In this situation the liver is dark green in colour and firm to the palpating probe.

Situations are encountered where it may be difficult to ascertain whether the gallbladder is more tense than normal. In these cases defective gallbladder emptying cannot be excluded by palpation with the probe. The intravenous administration of either cholecystokinin or ceruletide will solve this problem as either of these agents will induce vigorous contraction and emptying of the gallbladder in the normal individual.

Acute inflammation

In *acute obstructive cholecystitis*, which accounts for 85–90% of acutely inflamed gallbladders, the viscus appears tense and oedematous, with marked vascular injection which imparts a pinkish-red appearance. The omentum is often adherent to the fundus and *should not be teased from it* as it may be covering a sealed localized perforation or gangrenous patch. The latter are seen as dull greenish patches, usually in the region of the fundus.

Acute acalculous cholecystitis, which is usually encountered in the critically ill, has a similar laparoscopic appearance except that close inspection often reveals areas of infarction; the incidence of frank perforation of the gallbladder is higher than in the acute obstructive variety. The worse type of acute cholecystitis is the *emphysematous variety*, where the gallbladder has a swollen dusky appearance and crepitus of its walls can be elicited with the palpating probe. The condition affects the elderly and diabetics and is due to a mixed infection, including gas-forming anaerobes.

The laparoscopic appearance of an *empyema of the gallbladder* are distinctive: the organ is considerably enlarged, distended and creamy white with cyanotic dusky patches and adhesions to adjacent structures including omentum. By contrast a *mucocele of the gallbladder* appears as a large white tense viscus without any discolouration or evidence of inflammation.

Chronic inflammation

The laparoscopic findings in chronic cholecystitis are extremely variable and range from the fibrotic gallbladder (a whitish shrunken structure on the undersurface of the right lobe) to a thickened organ with opaque white walls and dense adhesions to surrounding structures. At times the gallbladder is not visible, being surrounded by omental adhesions involving, in addition, the liver and duodenum. The porcelain gallbladder (calcified fibrotic organ) is identified by tapping with the palpating probe.

Cholelithiasis

Gallstones may be detected by their impression through the gallbladder wall. They can also be palpated with the probe or detected by the ultrasound probe introduced through the accessory cannula.

Diverticula

True or congenital diverticula of the gallbladder are rare. At laparoscopy they appear as outpouchings of the fundus. Pseudo-diverticula are much more common and represent dilated Rokitans-ky–Aschoff sinuses (cholecystitis glandularis proliferans, adenomy-omatosis). A gallbladder harbouring these pseudodiverticula is usually observed at laparoscopy to be chronically inflamed, with thickened whitish walls and adhesions.

Carcinoma

Laparoscopy is the best method of detecting carcinoma of the gallbladder particularly at its early operable stage.[8] The lesion most commonly originates in the fundus and the appearance varies from a thickened plaque with neovasculature around its periphery to a large lobulated mass. Direct involvement of the right lobe by the tumour and hepatic deposits are readily identified. Thus laparoscopy, besides establishing the diagnosis, also indicates the need or otherwise for surgical intervention. Fine-needle cytology of the tumour mass or of the aspirated bile is used to confirm the diagnosis although the gross appearances of the advanced disease are unmistakable.

LIVER

The gross laparoscopic appearances of hepatic disorders are distinctive and often allow an experienced laparoscopist to make a diagnosis on the findings alone. However, forceps biopsy for exophytic lesions and needle core biopsy for flat lesions or diffuse disease should always be undertaken. Laparoscopic target liver biopsy is both safer and has a higher diagnostic yield than blind percutaneous biopsy.[9–13] The use of the palpating probe is essential, to visualize the posterior parts of the superior surface and the inferior surface of the liver.

Normal appearance

With the use of the palpating probe, only the posterior surface (pars affixa) is not visible by laparoscopy. The normal liver varies considerably in size. It has a reddish-brown colouration, the intensity of which varies depending on local blood perfusion (Plate 1). In addition the normal liver blanches readily on compression with the palpating probe. The colour of the liver tends to become darker with age due to the deposition of lipofuscin. In consistency, the normal liver is soft and pliable and tends to flop when elevated by the palpating probe. Its surface is smooth and glistening, reflecting the light in a uniform fashion. Some surface wrinkling and irregularity is observed in the elderly. The normal Glisson's capsule is thin and transparent and its blood and lymph vessels are not visible except with magnification and close inspection.

Congenital anomalies

These include (a) separation of the round ligament from the falciform ligament, which are normally contiguous and inserted together into the lobar fissure, (b) fenestrated falciform ligament, (c) anomalous segmentation of the right and left lobes and (d) the 'monkey' fissure, which results from parenchymal atrophy of the edge of the right lobe over the gallbladder. Riedel's lobe is common and consists of a tongue-like prolongation of the right lobe medial to the gallbladder. It is often mistaken clinically for a hepatic mass. Zahn's indentations consist of longitudinal furrowings on the anterosuperior surface of the liver and are thought to result from repeated pressure by the overlying diaphragmatic muscle bundles.

Cholestasis

With lower-power magnification the surface of the liver in both intra- and extrahepatic cholestasis appears uniformly light to dark green. However, on close inspection with magnification, a mottled appearance due to green spotting amidst the normal reddish-brown parenchyma is clearly visible. In mild cholestasis the normal liver colouration is seen with the low-power view: the green spotting, which tends to accentuate the normal surface texture, becomes evident only on close inspection and magnification.

Fatty change

This results in enlargement and blunting of the anterior margins which become swollen and rounded and a pale-coloured liver. The process starts as a lobular fatty change where on close inspection, the liver surface appears honeycombed with yellowish hexagonals outlined by orange-red margins, not dissimilar to a leopard's skin.[13] In the more advanced diffuse fatty infiltration the liver appears swollen and diffusely yellowish-orange. The laparoscopic appearances of a fatty liver give no indication as to the causative agent, so a target biopsy is essential.

Siderosis

This results from iron deposition in the liver caused by haemolysis, multiple blood transfusion etc. or may accompany postnecrotic cirrhosis, when its laparoscopic appearances and liver histology are virtually indistinguishable from those of haemochromatosis. The siderosis imparts a dark brown colouration to the liver whether it is cirrhotic or not.

Peliosis hepatis

This consists of irregular dark streaks beneath Glisson's capsule due to pooling of blood[14] and is found in severe fatty change of the liver, particularly after alcoholic intoxication, with lymphogranulomatosis, with hepatic neoplasms and following irradiation and systemic chemotherapy for malignant disease.

Acute hepatitis

Acute viral hepatitis *is not* an indication for laparoscopy and the diagnosis is usually established by the clinical features, laboratory and serological tests. However, on occasion, the diagnosis is missed and the patient may be subjected to emergency laparoscopy because of unexplained malaise and abdominal pain. In such a situation it is important that the condition is recognized and the necessary precautions taken to avoid spread of the hepatitis virus. The only case ever seen by one of the authors at laparoscopy was very distinctive. The liver appeared intensely red with an inflamed, glistening and oedematous appearance and rounded liver margin. Areas of fibrinous exudate and necrotic patches were visible on the anterosuperior surface and the normal liver surface pattern was lost.

Chronic persistent hepatitis

The laparoscopic appearances of this condition are largely nondescript. The liver has a brighter colour than usual, the edges are well defined and the gallbladder may be enlarged. Close inspection of the liver surface reveals a dense network of lymph vessels but the normal parenchymal pattern is retained. There is also some clouding of the capsule, but overt fibrosis is absent. The diagnosis and differentiation from the more serious chronic aggressive hepatitis requires a liver biopsy.

Chronic aggressive hepatitis

The liver appears more diseased, with obvious surface lymphangiectasis, capsular fibrosis and areas of necrosis. Atrophy of the left lobe may be present. Regenerative nodules with progression to cirrhosis are often present, together with postnecrotic scar fissuring which may separate the liver parenchyma into several 'lobular' and roundish masses (potato liver). Again a liver biopsy is essential to establish the diagnosis.

Sclerosing cholangitis

The laparoscopic appearances of primary and secondary sclerosing cholangitis are essentially identical. The liver appears inflamed, with a red colouration and is studded with green spots. The surface vascularity is increased. Small pitted scars resulting from the resolution of intrahepatic abscesses are often present. Capsular adhesions to the diaphragm and thickening of the Glisson's capsule may be encountered. The diagnosis of sclerosing cholangitis is, however, difficult and requires contrast radiology, liver biopsy and serological testing. The laparoscopic appearances cannot be relied upon for a definitive diagnosis.

Cirrhosis

There is no other diagnostic modality which approximates to the diagnostic potential of laparoscopy for the detection of cirrhosis of the liver since the procedure clearly shows the abnormal surface appearances of the disease: the scarring, regenerative nodules and the enlarged gallbladder.[15-17] In addition, laparoscopy can detect complications resulting from the disease: ascites, portal hypertension with splenomegaly and the development of hepatocellular carcinoma.

Contrary to often reiterated statements made by hepatologists who are not familiar with laparoscopy, the carcinomas developing in cirrhotic livers *rarely form large tumour masses* and are therefore often missed by CT scanning and other non-invasive modalities (Plates 5 and 6). The most common appearance of a carcinoma in a cirrhotic liver is a whitish elevated area of tissue among the darker regenerative nodules. Much less commonly, the neoplastic focus appears green. The tumour tends to be multicentric. These suspicious areas should be biopsied with the fine-pointed biopsy forceps (see Chapter 7).

It is customary to classify cirrhosis into micro- and macronodular varieties. Having witnessed a large series of cirrhotic livers through the laparoscope over a period of 20 years, we have been so impressed with the extreme variation in size of the regenerating nodules within a single liver as to doubt the validity of the classification into micro- and macronodular cirrhosis. Aetiological implications of the cirrhosis on the basis of the nodular size are therefore unsound. Very large nodules with dense fibrosis are, however, indicative of postnecrotic cirrhosis irrespective of aetiology.

Close inspection of the surface of the liver nodules reveals a surface granularity due to thickening of the Glisson's capsule and dilated lymphatics which may form multiple lymph cysts. The latter appear as whitish spots which may mimic a tuberculous miliary process.

Primary chronic nonsuppurative distinctive cholangitis–primary biliary cirrhosis

In the early non-cirrhotic stage of the disease, the laparoscopic appearances are those of an enlarged inflamed liver with an orange–red surface pattern and prominent surface vessels. As such, the condition cannot be diagnosed by the macroscopic appearance alone: deep core biopsies, preferably two or three from different areas of the liver, are necessary for histological examination, the findings of which are correlated with the results of the serological tests.[18]

The cirrhotic stage is easy to diagnose. The regenerating nodules are dark green at the top and become whitish as they merge with the surrounding thickened fibrotic capsule, which has prominent blood vessels and dilated lymphatics. The laparoscopic appearances of secondary biliary cirrhosis, resulting from chronic extrahepatic obstruction, are indistinguishable from those of the primary variety.

Portal hypertension

Dramatic visualization of the collateral circulation (Plate 9) can be obtained by laparoscopy in patients with portal hypertension. The changes include large tortuous distended veins which appear dark blue, from desaturated blood, networks of fine blood vessels in the subserosal planes (parietal peritoneum, undersurface of diaphragm, lienocolic and falciform ligaments), splenomegaly and an abnormal liver, with fibrosis, cirrhosis and congestion. In addition, ascites is usually present.

The large tortuous distended veins in the greater omentum are pathognomonic. Sometimes the para-umbilical veins become extremely dilated, with a bunched-up appearance, and can communicate with the left branch of the portal vein via the teres ligament; this is the Cruveilhier–Baumgarten syndrome.

In the Budd–Chiari syndrome and in veno-occlusive disease the liver is markedly enlarged and has a deep purplish, almost violaceous appearance, with areas of bluish discolouration and greatly distended and tortuous lymphatics. However, the liver surface remains smooth, and in this respect it differs from the passive venous congestion associated with congestive cardiac failure, where the surface is irregular and the liver shows a bluish–brown discolouration.

Laparoscopic splenoportography, although safe and well documented[12,13] is rarely used nowadays, especially since the advent of percutaneous transhepatic cannulation of the portal vein and its branches.

Liver cysts

Cystic lesions are well demonstrated by laparoscopy, they include solitary non-parasitic cysts, polycystic disease of the liver, Caroli's disease and parasitic cysts.[19]

Solitary non-parasitic cysts appear as smooth surface swellings with thin transparent walls. They contain either clear fluid, and so appear white, or bile-stained fluid, which imparts an amber discolouration and implies a possible communication with the biliary tract. Such amber-coloured cysts should not be aspirated during laparoscopy as this procedure may lead to bile leakage and peritonitis. Some long-standing large cysts may produce adhesions, presumably as a result of secondary infection.

In polycystic disease, the liver is studded by multiple water-clear cysts of varying sizes. The intervening hepatic parenchyma is normal. We have viewed only one case of Caroli's disease through the laparoscope. The Glisson's capsule was thickened and studded with several small dark green cysts. A laparoscopic biopsy of this patient showed features of both congenital cystic disease and congenital hepatic fibrosis. The endoscopic retrograde cholangiogram confirmed the laparoscopic appearances.

Hydatid cysts form large thick-walled round lesions and are creamy white in colour. They are usually surrounded by adhesions to adjacent structures and are more commonly encountered in the right lobe. The cystic nature of the lesion is confirmed by pressure with the palpating probe, unless the cyst is calcified. In that case, a gritty sensation is obtained and plain X-rays outline the calcified cystic lesion.

THE SPLEEN

The normal-sized spleen is covered with omentum and cannot be seen when the peritoneal cavity is inspected in the supine position. For laparoscopic inspection, the patient has to be turned on the right side with the head well elevated in the reversed Trendelenburg position. The palpating probe is used to tease away any residual omentum which does not fall away from the organ with this positional change. If the spleen is immediately visible in the supine position it must be enlarged.[20]

Accessory spleens constitute the most common congenital anomaly and are seen as spherical masses, 1–5 cm in diameter, usually near the lower pole or lateral to the spleen. Sometimes, deep indentations on the medial border appear to cut off a triangular segment from the main organ.

The changes that can be seen at laparoscopic examination include splenic enlargement from any cause, non-specific perisplenitis, gross thickening of the splenic capsule, nodular lesions in tuberculosis, Hodgkin's disease and sarcoidosis, splenic atrophy and splenic trauma. Although some advocate laparoscopic splenic needle biopsy,[21] this procedure is hazardous and should not be undertaken lightly: the incidence of bleeding after the procedure is considerable. Fortunately, with adequate bed rest, monitoring and blood transfusion, the need for surgical intervention to deal with continued life-threatening bleeding is rare.

The most striking splenic abnormality seen using laparoscopy is the sugar-icing spleen encountered in patients with congestive cardiac failure. The spleen appears white owing to gross thickening and hyaline change of the splenic capsule.

ASCITES

Ascites, which is visible as fluid in the paracolic gutters and pelvis, is detected by laparoscopy before it can be diagnosed by other means.

In the majority of patients the aetiology of the ascites can be obtained by clinical and laboratory assessment including cytological examination of a sample of the ascitic fluid. In this respect, it is important to stress that in ascites the intestines float on the surface of the fluid and are therefore liable to be damaged by blind percutaneous sampling of ascitic fluid unless special precautions are taken: the aspiration is done laterally in an area of obvious dullness to percussion. Laparoscopy is generally reserved for those patients in whom the aetiology cannot be ascertained by less invasive methods.[22]

In gross ascites, the intra-abdominal pressure is raised and the amount of gas required to inflate the peritoneal cavity prior to laparoscopic inspection is much smaller (about one litre) than usual. It will be difficult to study the peritoneal cavity if there are substantial amounts of ascitic fluid. In this case, removal of about 500 ml of the fluid via the suction cannula is necessary. Provided this is done slowly, no untoward reactions will be encountered. Placing the patient in the reversed Trendelenburg position will change the position of the fluid level, improving the view of the liver lobes.

The macroscopic fluid observed at laparoscopy often indicates the nature of the underlying disease and can be classified as serous (yellow/green), chylous, pseudochylous, blood-stained, or myxomatous (colloidal).

Ascites in liver disease

In cirrhosis the ascitic fluid is usually clear, yellow to green and frothy (Plate 2). Cirrhotic and portal hypertensive changes are also evident at laparoscopy. In long-standing cirrhotic ascites the fluid becomes opalescent and/or turbid (pseudochylous) as a result of changes in the protein constituents; it then resembles and has to be differentiated from chylous ascites which is caused by lymphatic obstruction.

Ascites in inflammatory disease

This is usually serous and yellow and is encountered in tuberculous peritonitis and Crohn's disease. In addition to the ascitic fluid, miliary tubercles are seen on the peritoneal surfaces of the parietes and viscera. However, these may be difficult to distinguish from other miliary foci such as sarcoidosis and multiple tumour deposits and biopsies are essential. Specimens are obtained for both culture and histology. In Crohn's disease, the inflamed bowel with thickening, congestion and oedema of the bowel wall and the foreshortening of the mesentery are obvious.

Ascites in malignant disease

The macroscopic appearances of the fluid varies considerably. It may be clear and yellow, dark green in malignant bile duct obstruction, chylous as a result of malignant obstruction of the lymphatic channels, frankly blood-stained and gelatinous or mucinous. The latter is encountered in some instances of primary mesothelioma of the peritoneum, in secondary deposits from some ovarian carcinomas and less commonly in pseudomucinous carcinoma of the appendix. The appearance is that of accumulations of gelatinous material adherent to bowel loops and the parietes. In some instances clear mucinous masses hang from the peritoneal cavity like collections of frogspawn.

Multiple tumour nodules may be seen on both visceral and parietal peritoneum and on the greater omentum. When the latter is heavily involved, it becomes rolled up and forms a hard mass of malignant tissue. Biopsy of the lesions with the fine-pointed forceps is essential for confirmation.

Chylous ascites is distinguished by its milky appearance, on biochemical analysis it is found to have a high fat content. It indicates lymphatic obstruction due to intestinal lymphangiectasis, lymphoma or extensive nodal deposits from carcinoma.

Ascites due to chronic congestive cardiac disease

This is usually encountered in constrictive pericarditis and tricuspid incompetence. In addition to the granular congested dark brown liver, a yellowish-brown turbid fluid is encountered. The spleen is also enlarged as a result of chronic congestion and may have a white appearance due to gross thickening of the splenic capsule. It is important that the laparoscopic stab wounds are closed adequately by full-thickness abdominal wall sutures to avoid leakage of ascitic fluid, which is a source of great inconvenience to these patients.

REFERENCES

1 Cuschieri, A. (1975) Value of laparoscopy in hepatobiliary disease. *Ann. R. Coll. Surg. 57:* 33–38.
2 Kimura, R.K., Wakui, K., Ishioka, K. et al. (1976) Significance of peritoneoscopic examination, direct cholangiography and cytological examination of aspirated bile in the diagnosis of biliary and pancreatic malignancies. *Tohoku J. exp. Med. (Suppl.), 118:* 145–148.
3 Look, D., Henning, H. & Yano, M. (1975) Direkte Ultraschallechographie der Gallenblase unter laparoskopischer Sicht. In *Fortschritte der gastroenterologischen Endoskopie, Bd. 6.,* Linder, H. Baden-Baden: Witzstrock.

4   Fukuda, M., Mima, S., Tarrabe, T. et al. (1984) Endoscopic sonography of the liver–diagnostic application of the echolaparoscope to localize intrahepatic lesions. *Scand. J. Gastroenterol. (Suppl.),* 102: 24–38.
5   Frank, K., Bliesze, H., Beck, K. et al. (1983) Laparoscopic sonography. A new dimension in the diagnostic approach to internal organs. *Dt. med. Wschr.* 108: 902–904.
6   Okita, K., Kodama, T., Oda, M. & Takemoto, T. (1984) Laparoscopic ultrasonography. Diagnosis of liver and pancreatic cancer. *Scand. J. Gastroenterol. (Suppl.),* 94: 91–100.
7   Ohta, Y. (1983) New ultrasonic laparoscope for diagnosis of intra-abdominal diseases. *Gastrointest. Endosc. 28:* 233–239.
8   Bhargava, D.K., Sarin, S., Varma, K. & Kapur, B.M. (1983) Laparoscopy in carcinoma of the gallbladder. *Gastrointest. Endosc. 29:* 21–22.
9   Friedman, I.H. & Wolff, W.I. (1977) Laparoscopy. A safe method for liver biopsy in the high risk patient. *Am. J. Gastroenterol. 67:* 319–323.
10 Trujillo, N.P. (1976) Peritoneoscopy and guided biopsy in the diagnosis of intra-abdominal disease. *Gastroenterology, 71:* 1083–1085.
11 Jori, G.P. & Peschle, C. (1972) Combined peritoneoscopy and liver biopsy in the diagnosis of hepatic neoplasm. *Gastroenterology, 63:* 1016–1019.
12 Conn, H.O. (1972) Percutaneous versus peritoneoscopic liver biopsy. *Gastroenterology, 63:* 1074–1075.
13 Beck, K. (1984) *Color Atlas of Laparoscopy.* Philadelphia: Saunders.
14 Solis-Herruzo, J.A. (1983) Reddish-purple areas on the liver surface: the laparoscopic picture of peliosis hepatis. *Endoscopy, 15:* 96–100.
15 Henning, H. (1983) Diagnostic procedures in the evaluation of hepatic disease. Laparoscopy. *Lab. Res. Methods biol. Med. 7:* 469–488.
16 Editorial (1978) Use of laparoscopy in liver disease. *Br. med. J. i:* 738–739.
17 Girard, M., Coulot, M. & Hallacq, A. (1960) Diagnostic importance of peritoneoscopy in liver cirrhosis. *J. méd. Lyon, 41:* 153–159.
18 Linder, H.R., Dammermann, G. & Klöppel, G. (1977) The laparoscopic staging of primary biliary cirrhosis. *Endoscopy, 9:* 68–70.
19 Banche, M., Ferrari, A. & Roatta, L. (1975) Il ruolo della laparoscopia nella diagnosi delle formazioni cistiche del fegato. *Minerva gastroent. 21:* 45–47.
20 Mullier, J.P., Kadende, P., Burette, A. et al. (1981) The spleen at laparoscopy. Clinical, scintigraphic and endoscopic correlations. *Acta gastro-enterol. belg. 44:* 187–194.
21 Dagnini, G., Cladironi, M.W., Marin, G. & Paletta, M. (1984) Laparoscopic splenic biopsy. *Endoscopy, 16:* 55–58.
22 Cunningham, J.T. (1982) Peritoneoscopy: use in the diagnosis of ascites of unknown origin. *J. Scott. med. Assoc. 78:* 269–273.
23 McCallum, R.W. & Berci, G. (1976) Laparoscopy in hepatic disease. *Gastrointest. Endosc. 23:* 20–24.
24 Berci, G., Shore, J.M., Morgenstern, L.M. & Shapiro, S. (1973) A direct approach to the differential diagnosis of jaundice. *Am. J. Surg. 126:* 577–586.

9
Interventional Laparoscopy

This important aspect of laparoscopy is practised by only a few surgeons and gastroenterologists. It is a well established procedure in obstetrics and gynaecology, e.g. for retrieval of ova for in-vitro fortilization and laparoscopic sterilization, for example (see Chapter 12). Interventional laparoscopy is attended by an increased risk of complications and should be attempted only by those who are experienced with diagnostic laparoscopy. In expert hands and with strict adherence to certain essential requirements, interventional laparoscopy is safe. The need for emergency surgical intervention to deal with a life-threatening complication has arisen only once in 150 cases of interventional laparoscopy by the author.

It is perhaps in this area that future developments of laparoscopy will be realized, and the advent of ultrasonic probes and guided laser beams opens a new field for diagnostic and therapeutic purposes.

REQUIREMENTS FOR INTERVENTIONAL LAPAROSCOPY

1   Careful preoperative assessment is necessary. This entails a full clotting profile in jaundiced patients. All patients undergoing interventional laparoscopy should be blood-grouped and cross-matched with a minimum of two units of blood.
2   Interventional laparoscopy should only be undertaken within the confines of an operating theatre suite with patient monitoring both during and after the procedure.
3   All patients must be kept in bed for at least 12 hours after the procedure, with a minimum of one overnight stay in hospital.
4   The procedure should be performed under general anaesthesia with endotracheal intubation and muscle relaxants.
5   The urinary bladder should be catheterized prior to the procedure and the catheter connected to a drainage bag.
6   A diathermy pad adequately connected to the diathermy machine is placed beneath the buttocks of the patient.
7   Peritoneal insufflation must always be with CO_2 since diathermy may be used during the procedure.
8   Accessory instruments and appropriate trocars for the procedure to be undertaken must be available.

9   An assistant is necessary in addition to the scrub nurse. In this situation a teaching attachment, which is fitted to the telescope and which allows both the operator and the assistant simultaneous views of the intraperitoneal field, greatly facilitates the procedure.

LAPAROSCOPIC CHOLANGIOGRAPHY

This can be performed either trans-hepatically or transcystically, if the gallbladder is present. For the former approach, the Chiba needle is used, whereas the sheathed Longdwel needle is preferable for the transcystic approach. In either case, the anaesthetized patient is placed on an X-ray operating table and the image intensifier is connected and switched on ready for use. After insufflation of the peritoneal cavity with CO_2, a preliminary inspection of the abdominal cavity and liver is carried out. The appropriate site of insertion of the cholangiography needle is ascertained by finger depression of the abdominal wall beneath the right costal margin whilst viewing the indented region through the telescope.

Trans-hepatic cholangiography

The Chiba needle is introduced into the substance of the right lobe just medial to the gallbladder on the anterosuperior surface of the liver some 5 cm from the anterior edge, to a depth of approximately 5 cm, and directed inferomedially. The Chiba needle is then connected by a PVC tube and a three-way tap to two 30 ml syringes, one containing 20% Hypaque (sodium diatrizoate) and the other, normal saline. Screening is commenced as small increments of 1–2 ml of contrast are injected. When the needle tip is inside a vascular channel, contrast is seen to disappear readily in a centrifugal direction. The needle is withdrawn 0.5 cm and the contrast injection repeated. The procedure continues until the image clearly shows that the needle is in the ductal system, with retention of the contrast in a clearly defined tubular structure. At this stage a further 20 ml are injected slowly and if the biliary tree is outlined on the image intensifier, films are taken for permanent record (Figure 9.1). The amount of contrast needed to obtain adequate visualization of the entire biliary tract varies with the extent of dilatation of the intra-hepatic biliary tree. Occasionally, up to 60 ml may be required.

Pitfalls

1   The needle may be inserted too deeply so that it penetrates right through the hepatic substance to emerge on the postero-inferior

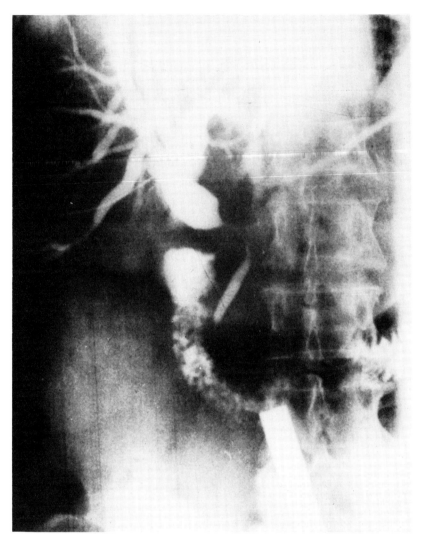

Fig. 9.1 Laparoscopic trans-hepatic cholangiogram showing bile duct obstruction by a pancreatic neoplasm.

surface. This becomes immediately apparent when contrast is injected. Withdrawal of the needle by about 1 cm is the required remedial action.

2 The needle tip may be in the hepatic parenchyma outside a vascular or biliary channel. This is recognized when injection produces a blob of contrast which accumulates around the needle tip.

Whenever this happens no further contrast is injected until the needle has been withdrawn a further 0.5–1.0 cm.

3 Bleeding or bile leak from the needle puncture on withdrawal of the needle is usually stopped by pressure on the area by the palpating probe, which is introduced in the left hypochondrium through an accessory cannula.

Trans-cystic cholangiography

This is a well established and reliable technique[1–4] and is indicated in jaundiced patients with an intact gallbladder undergoing laparoscopy. The sheathed Longdwel needle is ideally suited for this procedure. The principle of this safe technique is to enter the gallbladder through the edge of the right lobe and gallbladder fossa (Figure 9.2). On subsequent removal of the cannula, the tamponade effect of the liver substance prevents bile leakage. On no account should the gallbladder be punctured directly as bile will leak from the puncture site into the peritoneal cavity after the procedure.

The procedure is performed as follows. The optimal site of entry of the sheathed needle over the edge of the right lobe overhanging the gallbladder fundus is ascertained by indenting the abdominal wall

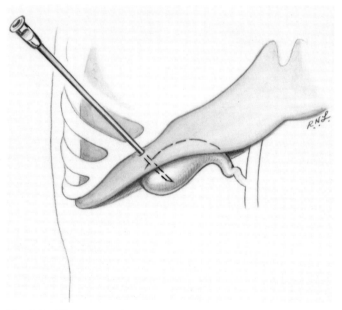

Fig. 9.2 Diagrammatic representation of the technique of trans-cystic cholangiography. The sheathed Longdwel needle is inserted through the edge of the right lobe and the gallbladder fossa into the lumen of the organ.

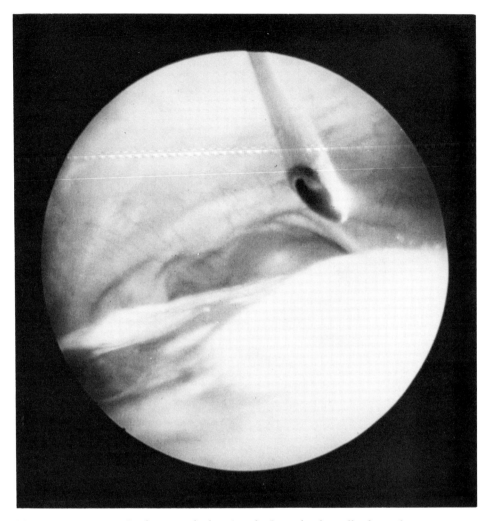

Fig. 9.3 Laparoscopic photograph showing the Longdwel needle above the edge of the right lobe.

while viewing with the telescope. The needle assembly is then inserted through the abdominal wall into the peritoneal cavity under visual control (Figure 9.3) and the needle tip is then guided to enter the right lobe some 1–2 cm from the edge of the liver at a point which approximates to the centre of the gallbladder fossa. The anaesthetist is asked to stop ventilation momentarily as the needle is transversing the liver substance. Continued *controlled* pressure on the needle assembly results in a sudden give. This signifies that the needle tip

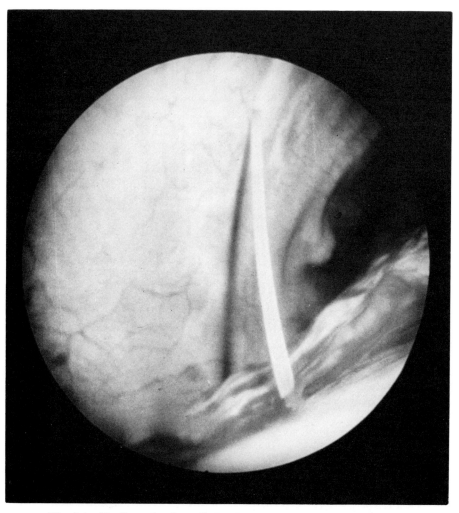

Fig. 9.4 The Longdwel needle has been inserted into the gallbladder lumen and the metal needle removed, leaving the outer sheath in situ. Before injection, trial aspiration for bile is carried out.

has entered the gallbladder lumen. At this point the shaft of the needle assembly is advanced a further 0.5 cm. The inner metal section of the assembly is then withdrawn leaving the outer PVC sheath in situ (Figure 9.4). A syringe is then applied to the female Luer fitting, and on aspiration bile should be obtained. A three-way tap connected to two 30 ml syringes, one containing 20% Hypaque and the other physiological saline, is fitted to the sheath. The operating table is tilted head down approximately 30° and contrast injection is started

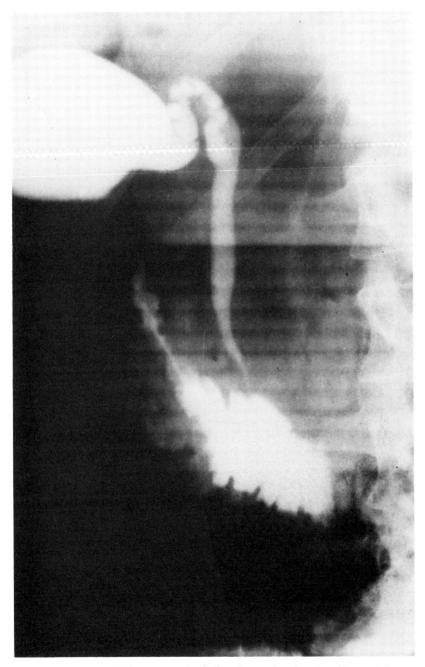

Fig. 9.5 Trans-cystic laparoscopic cholangiography showing filling of the gallbladder.

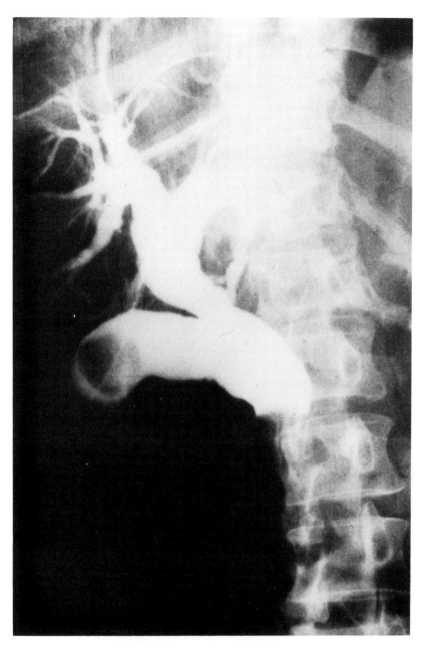

Fig. 9.6   Trans-cystic laparoscopic cholangiogram showing large bile duct obstruction due to a stone impacted at the lower end of the common bile duct.

with simultaneous image intensification. Usually 20–30 ml are required to fill the gallbladder before the contrast begins to drain from the organ via the cystic duct into the common bile duct (Figure 9.5). The amount of contrast required to outline the biliary tract will vary according to the extent of dilatation. In general, however, a further injection of 20–30 ml of contrast is necessary (Figure 9.6). At the end of the procedure, the gallbladder is aspirated via the sheath until it is seen through the laparoscope to have collapsed; the sheath is then withdrawn.

Pitfalls

1   The needle may be inserted too near to the liver edge, so that the needle tip misses the gallbladder. The needle is withdrawn and reinserted into the hepatic substance directing its tip to the centre of the gallbladder fossa.

2   The needle tip may not be inserted far enough, so that the end of the needle assembly lies in the gallbladder fossa outside the gallbladder lumen. This becomes apparent when bile is not obtained during trial aspiration. If this occurs the inner metal shaft is re-introduced inside the sheath and the tip of the entire assembly is advanced further under laparoscopic guidance. The inner metal needle is then withdrawn and trial aspiration is repeated.

3   *Perforation of the gallbladder* can happen if the entry of the needle into the gallbladder is not performed under visual control; it is therefore preventable. It results from over-advancement of the needle, such that it traverses the gallbladder lumen and then penetrates its inferior wall. If perforation should occur, the needle assembly should be withdrawn slowly until the tip disappears into the gallbladder. The inner needle is then removed and all bile is aspirated from the gallbladder under direct vision. Saline is then injected into the gallbladder until it distends again. The saline injection is continued until the extent of leakage from the perforation can be assessed. If this is minimal, the gallbladder is emptied by aspiration, a drain is inserted in the right subhepatic pouch and the procedure is terminated. The patient is put on systemic antibiotics and observed closely for the next 24 hours. Excessive leakage observed when the gallbladder is filled with saline warrants an immediate laparotomy and suture of the perforation.

LAPAROSCOPIC CHOLECYSTOSTOMY

This procedure was first introduced as an alternative means of laparoscopic preoperative decompression in patients severely jaundiced because of distal extra-hepatic biliary tract obstruction. With the

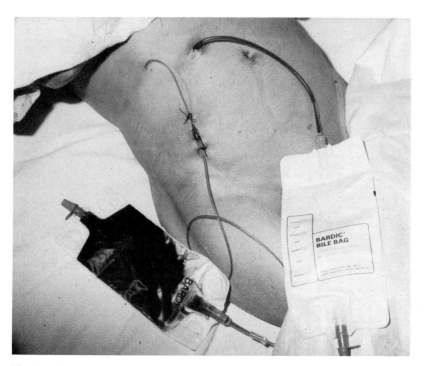

Fig. 9.7   Laparoscopic cholecystostomy. A pig-tail catheter is used to minimize the risk of dislodgement.

advent of transhepatic or endoscopic insertion of indwelling prostheses, the indication for the use of laparoscopic decompression has largely disappeared. The procedure has other therapeutic indications, particularly in symptomatic patients with gallstones or acute cholecystitis who are elderly or unfit for surgery by virtue of severe cardiorespiratory disease. The insertion of a percutaneous pig-tail catheter into the gallbladder readily drains a gallbladder distended as a result of acute obstructive cholecystitis, empyema or mucocele. In addition it provides ready access for stone dissolution by the local instillation of solvents.

The technique employed is similar to that used for trans-cystic cholangiography. A nephrostomy-type pig-tail catheter is used; it is introduced under laparoscopic guidance through the edge of the right lobe into the gallbladder lumen with the same precautions as outlined previously for trans-cystic cholangiography. The technique is particularly easy in patients with large distended gallbladders. The indwelling catheter is connected to a closed system of drainage (Figure 9.7). Following maturation of the cholecystostomy tract over a

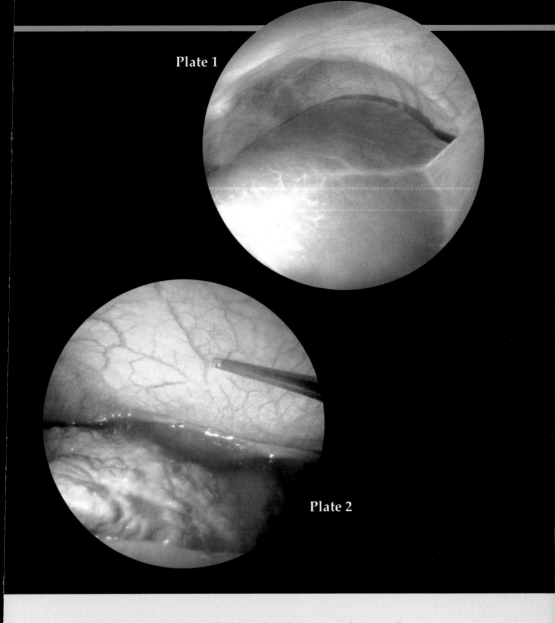

Plate 1 Normal-looking right lobe of the liver. Note the smooth appearance of the anterior surface. Fine vessels on the parietal peritoneum and falciform ligament are well seen. There is some surface scarring of the liver but this is within the normal range. With modern optics minute changes can be discovered from a distance and a large part of the organ can be seen.

Plate 2 Cirrhotic (left) lobe of liver, with ascitic fluid in the paracolic gutter. The suction coagulation probe points to enlarged veins on the parietal peritoneum, indicating the presence of portal hypertension.

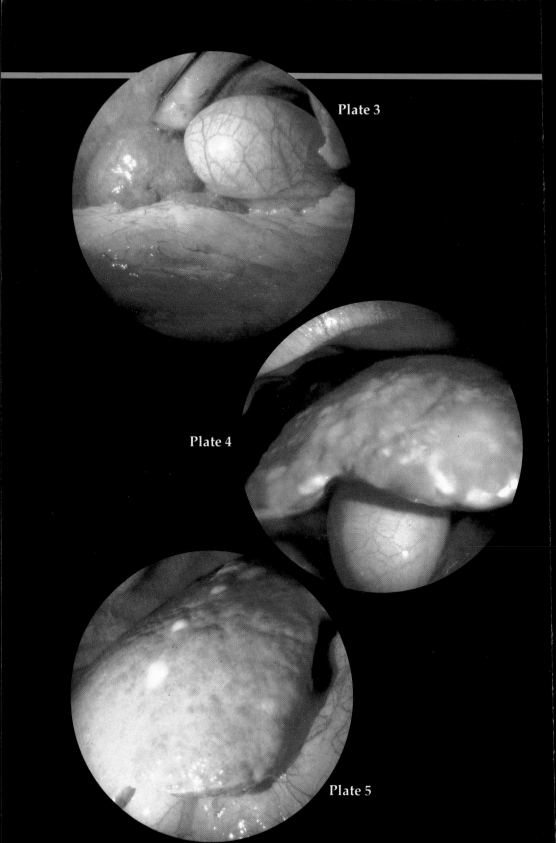

Plate 3

Plate 4

Plate 5

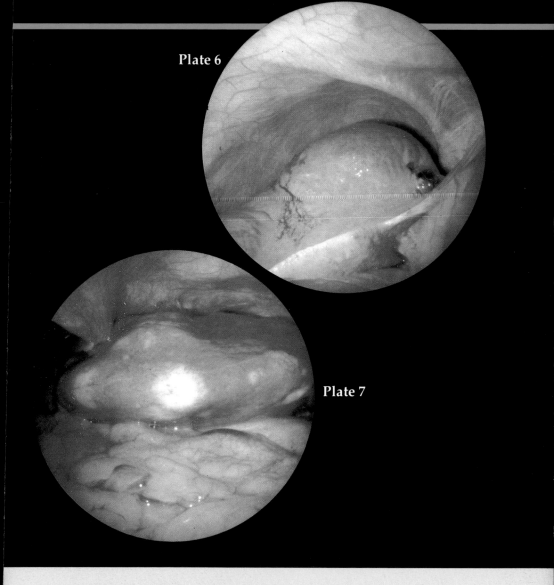

Plate 6

Plate 7

Plate 3   Shrunken cirrhotic right lobe of liver with palpation probe advanced above. Note the distended gallbladder.

Plate 4   Irregular surface of cirrhotic liver with the smooth but distended gallbladder which is commonly observed in cirrhotic patients.

Plate 5   Cirrhotic right lobe of liver with whitish protruding lesions which were not discovered by computed tomography or scintiscan. Biopsy showed hepatocellular carcinoma in cirrhotic liver parenchyma.

Plate 6   The asymmetry or protruding area of the right lobe (dome) of liver is immediately obvious. In these cases Tru-Cut needle biopsies of the suspicious areas are recommended. For details of biopsy technique see Chapter 7.

Plate 7   Metastatic lesions in left lobe of liver from a primary carcinoma of the left colon.

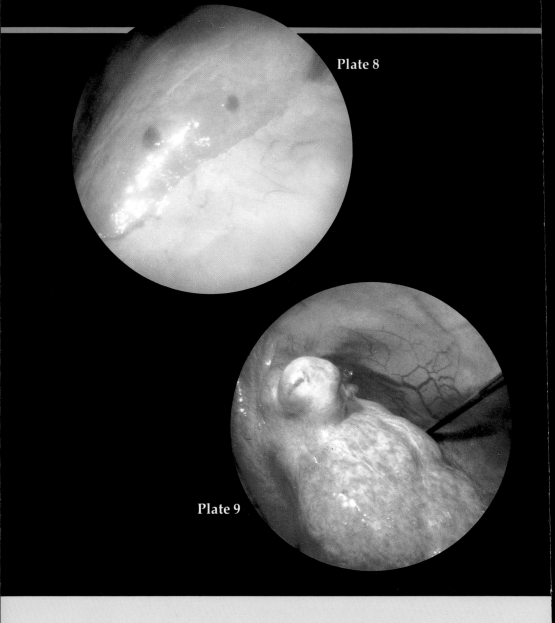

Plate 8   Metastatic melanoma in right lobe of liver. The primary lesion was on the trunk.

Plate 9   Irregular left lobe of liver, and enlarged veins on parietal peritoneum in a case of Budd–Chiari syndrome with venous cystic degeneration. Note protruding bluish area beside falciform ligament.

period of four weeks it is possible to withdraw the catheter and insert the Olympus fibre-optic choledochoscope (Figure 9.8) for inspection of the gallbladder lumen and stone extraction by means of the modified Dormia basket. Preliminary dilatation of the tract to a size of French gauge 16 with plastic dilators is necessary.

More potent solvents are now available, such as methyl tert-butyl ether (MTBE).[8] These are capable of achieving gallstone dissolution within hours of instillation. Laparoscopic cholecystostomy may be the best method of achieving gallstone dissolution by this method. More recently, extracorporeal shock-wave lithotripsy has been used to fragment gallstones.[9] Although the initial results are encouraging, the passage of the gallstone fragments has been a problem in some cases. In our opinion the use of laparoscopic cholecystostomy will provide a non-surgical and safe method for the removal of these fragments.

LAPAROSCOPIC ASSESSMENT OF THE PANCREAS AND FINE-NEEDLE ASPIRATION BIOPSY

There are two laparoscopic approaches which are used to visualize the pancreas. The supragastric method was first introduced by Meyer-Burg[5] in 1971 and the infragastric route by Strauch et al. in 1973.[6] The authors have used both methods in the management of patients with pancreatic cancer, where the technique is of unquestionable value in establishing a definitive diagnosis by guided fine-needle cytology and in staging the extent of the disease and therefore the necessity or otherwise for surgical intervention. In our experience laparoscopic assessment is more reliable than other diagnostic modalities such as ultrasound and CT scanning both in providing a definitive diagnosis and in the confirmation of advanced inoperable disease.[7]

Accessory instruments

In addition to the basic laparoscopy set, two accessory trocars, laparoscopic biopsy forceps, laparoscopic scissors, laparoscopic coagulation forceps, laparoscopic tubal grasping forceps, palpating probe and a fine Chiba needle (23G) are required.

Supragastric method (Figure 9.9)

This should be tried first as it is the easier of the two techniques and is particularly suitable in thin patients. After insufflation of the

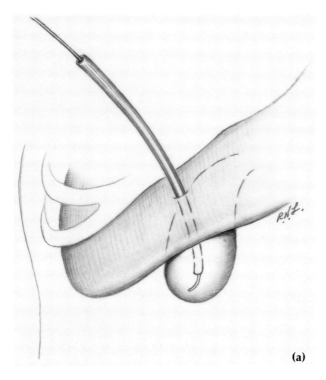

(a)

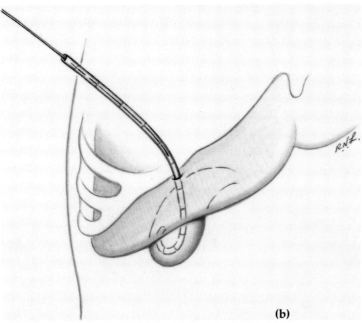

(b)

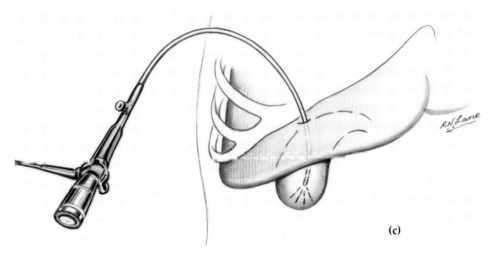

(c)

Fig. 9.8   (a) A guide wire is inserted into the gallbladder and the cholecystostomy catheter is removed. (b) The tract is dilated with graded plastic dilators to size 18 FG. (c) The flexible choledochoscope is then introduced and connected to a saline irrigation.

peritoneal cavity, a preliminary thorough inspection of the liver and peritoneum is performed to determine the presence or absence of metastatic disease. If present, laparoscopic biopsies are taken with the biopsy forceps. The first accessory trocar is inserted in the right hypochondrium under visual control. The palpating probe is introduced through it and is advanced under direct vision until it lies beneath the edge of the liver. The palpating probe is then used to elevate the liver to expose the gastrohepatic omentum. In thin patients the lesser omentum is so thin as to appear as a transparent film covering the pancreas, which can be seen clearly through it. More usually, however, the omentum is too fat for the pancreas to be visualized. At this stage the second accessory trocar is inserted in the left hypochrondrium under direct vision. Whilst the assistant lifts the edge of the liver with the palpating probe, the laparoscopic scissors are advanced and used to cut a small hole through an avascular area of the lesser omentum. At this stage the scissors are withdrawn and the palpating probe advanced into the hole in the lesser omentum. Downward pressure on the probe will enlarge the hole in the lesser omentum. The palpating probe is advanced further and used to elevate the liver substance. The telescope is then introduced into the lesser sac for inspection of the lesser sac. If bleeding is encountered from the edges of the opening in the lesser sac, this can easily be controlled by diathermy coagulation. *The opening in the lesser omentum*

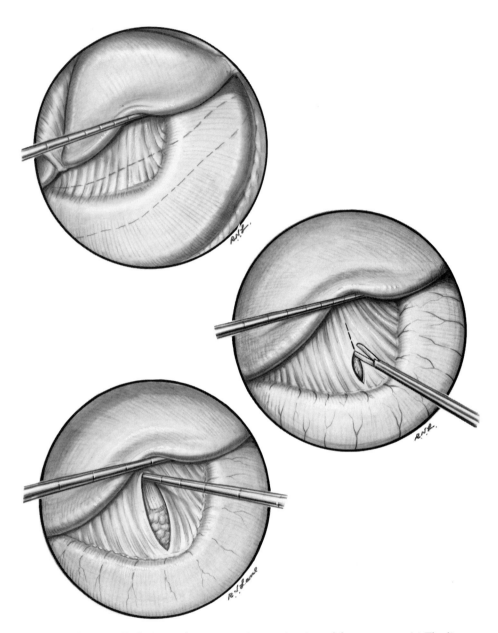

Fig. 9.9   Technique of supragastric examination of the pancreas. (a) The liver is elevated by the first palpating probe to expose the lesser omentum and lesser curvature of the stomach. (b) Through a second accessory cannula the laparoscopic scissors are used to cut a hole in an avascular area of the omentum. (c) The hole is enlarged by the second palpating probe and the telescope is then inserted into the lesser sac.

must be equidistant between the pylorus and the cardio-oesophageal junction and at least 2 cm from the lesser curvature of the stomach. This ensures penetration through a relatively avascular area and avoids injury to the right and left gastric vessels.

The limitations of the supragastric approach are twofold. Firstly, visualization of the body and tail is incomplete, particularly in those individuals with a short lesser omentum. Secondly, the procedure fails in about 30% of cases because of a greatly thickened fatty omentum or the presence of adhesions, particularly after cholecystectomy or surgery for peptic ulcer disease.

Infragastric method

This approach gives a better visualization of the lesser sac and body and tail of the pancreas than the supragastric method and is favoured by one of the authors except in very thin patients.

After insufflation and initial exploratory laparoscopy, the first accessory trocar is inserted along the lateral edge of the right rectus muscle 1–2 cm above the umbilicus and through it is introduced the tubal grasping forceps. This is used to grasp the gastro-colic omentum which is pulled downwards and held on the stretch. The second accessory trocar is inserted in the left upper quadrant half-way up the linea semilunaris (Figure 9.10). Through this is introduced the coagulation forceps and a few small vessels crossing one of the transparent windows in the gastro-colic omentum along the greater curvature are cauterized. The coagulation forceps is then replaced by the laparoscopic scissors and an opening is cut to gain access to the lesser sac adjacent to the greater curvature. The tubal grasping forceps is removed from the first accessory cannula and replaced by the palpating probe which is introduced under visual control through the opening in the gastrocolic omentum for a distance of 5 cm and then used to elevate the stomach. The telescope is then introduced into the lesser sac and inspection of the lesser sac, pancreas and splenic hilum commences (Figure 9.11). This procedure has been successfully performed by one of the authors without any complications in 65 patients. The success rate in pancreas visualization in the last 40 cases has been 85%. Failures are due to marked obesity and gross adhesions from previous surgery in the supracolic compartment.

FINE-NEEDLE CYTOLOGY OF THE PANCREAS

A fine 23 gauge Chiba needle attached to a 10 ml disposable syringe is used. Cell yield is considerably enhanced if the lumen of the needle is

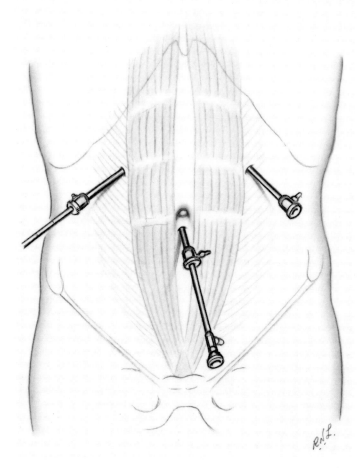

Fig. 9.10 Sites of insertion of the main and accessory trocars for infragastric examination of the pancreas. The main trocar is introduced through a subumbilical stab incision, the first accessory trocar along the left linea semilunaris above the umbilicus and the second accessory trocar through the equivalent site on the right side.

previously dipped in heparin solution (1000 units/ml), which is drawn in to the assembled needle–syringe and then squirted out.

The original method was to guide the needle into the lesser sac through the opening in the lesser or greater omentum. This, however, can be difficult with the telescope already in the lesser sac and the technique has been abandoned in favour of the transgastric approach. With this technique the fine Chiba needle penetrates the walls of the stomach and is then guided by the laparoscope into the pancreatic lesion. Suction by the syringe is maintained as the needle

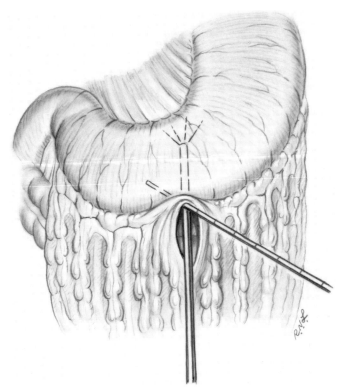

Fig. 9.11 Technique of infragastric examination of the pancreas. The palpating probe has been inserted through the opening in the gastro-colic omentum and used to elevate the greater curvature and posterior wall of the stomach from the pancreas. The telescope is then inserted into the lesser sac.

transverses the lesion in at least three directions over a period of 20–30 seconds. The needle is then withdrawn and immediate smears are prepared.

Preparation of smears

The Chiba needle is disconnected from the syringe and the plunger of the syringe is withdrawn up to the 10 ml mark. The needle, which is then re-attached to the syringe nozzle, is directed 1 cm above the centre of a previously labelled microscope glass slide and by forceful ejection, the material is squirted onto the slide (Figure 9.12). The procedure is repeated three times to obtain sufficient material for smears. Thereafter a second slide is laid on top of the first one and two squash preparations are made by sliding the top slide against the

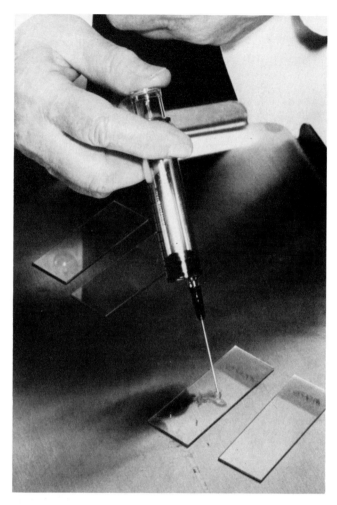

Fig. 9.12   The material obtained by aspiration is ejected onto an already labelled glass slide.

other (Figure 9.13). The residual material in the needle–syringe assembly is deposited into a container with fixative (Carbowax) by aspirating the fluid and re-injecting it into the container several times. This fluid is later centrifuged and further smears prepared from it.

Staining

One of the two fresh squash smears is stained immediately (with Diff Quik haematology stain) for reporting, ideally within five minutes

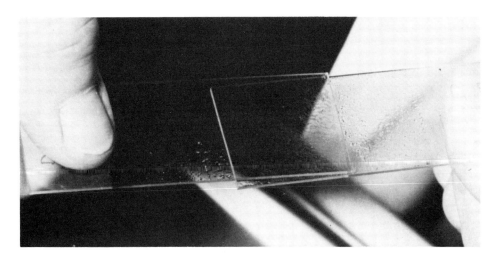

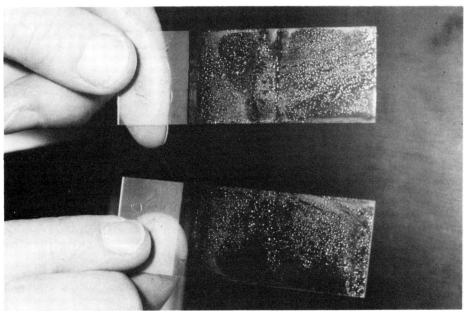

Fig. 9.13   Preparation of squash smears for pancreatic cytology.

(Figure 9.14). The other squash preparation is sprayed with a plastic spray and subsequently stained with Giemsa or Papanicolaou stain. The smears obtained from the centrifuged deposit of the carbowax fixative are stained with haematoxylin and eosin. The main advantage of the immediate Diff Quik stain is that it ensures an adequate cellular specimen has been obtained. This is especially

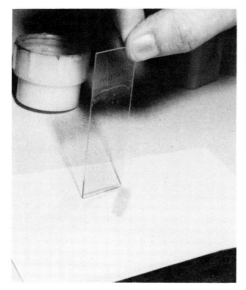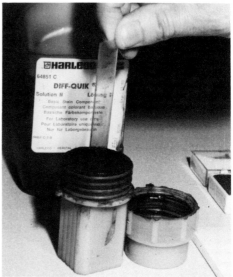

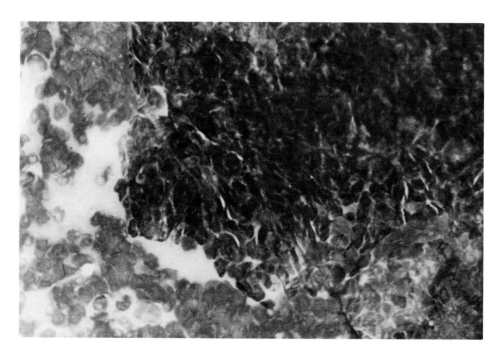

Fig. 9.14   Diff Quik staining of pancreatic cytology smear (top), showing malignant cells (bottom). With this staining technique a diagnosis is obtained four minutes after the procedure is performed.

useful during early training in fine-needle aspiration. If the smear is judged to be unsatisfactory because it contains few or no pancreatic acinar cells the procedure is repeated. Diff Quik staining also allows an immediate cytological diagnosis of the pancreatic lesions (Figure 9.14) and in our experience of 52 cases, the results of Diff Quik staining are very reliable and correlate well with those obtained by Giemsa and Papanicolaou staining.

LAPAROSCOPIC ADHESIOLYSIS

A group of patients, usually females, suffer from chronic abdominal pain after previous surgical intervention. Full investigation of these patients by the gastroenterologist is frequently negative and laparoscopy is often carried out to ascertain the cause of their pain.[10] In about 30% of these patients, laparoscopy confirms a pathology within the peritoneal cavity, for example gallstone disease, small bowel Crohn's disease, tubo-ovarian disease etc. One of the most common findings is the presence of significant adhesions to the abdominal parietes. In the absence of other pathology, we have undertaken laparoscopic adhesiolysis in these patients. Although assessment of the effects of laparoscopic enterolysis is essentially subjective, relief of pain was obtained in 20 out of 32 patients who underwent this procedure. Furthermore, laparoscopic adhesiolysis has not been accompanied by any complications.

Accessory instruments

In addition to the standard laparoscopic set, the following instruments are required: accessory trocar, palpating probe, laparoscopic coagulation forceps and laparoscopic scissors.

A diathermy pad is applied to the patient and its lead connected to the electrosurgical unit. The site of entry of the Veress needle and subsequent main trocar depends on the site of the previous operation scar (see Chapter 4). In principle, however, the entry site should be well away from such scars and preferably in a quadrant diametrically opposite. The abdomen is insufflated with CO_2 and the laparoscope is then introduced, after which a thorough inspection of the peritoneal cavity is performed. Particular attention is paid to the anatomy of the adhesions. The significant ones are those which are inserted into the anterior abdominal wall and connect with the omentum or small bowel. Fortunately these adhesions can be divided at laparoscopy with complete safety.

Technique

The accessory trocar is introduced along the linea semilunaris at the level of the umbilicus on the right or left side, depending on the exact anatomy and location of the adhesions. The coagulating forceps and the laparoscopic scissors are introduced through this accessory cannula. The technique involves division of the adhesion close to the anterior abdominal wall, since this is the least vascular part (Figure 9.15). Any bleeding encountered is arrested by diathermy. As the peritoneal cavity is fully insufflated the adhesions are stretched thereby facilitating their division. *Adequate insufflation of the peritoneal cavity with CO_2 is therefore essential for laparoscopic adhesiolysis* and the insufflation must keep the abdomen sufficiently tense throughout the procedure.

Afterwards, the patient is kept under observation on oral liquids only for the next 24 hours. Solid food is given after the patient has passed flatus. A minor degree of ileus lasting 1–2 days may be encountered in patients after extensive laparoscopic adhesiolysis.

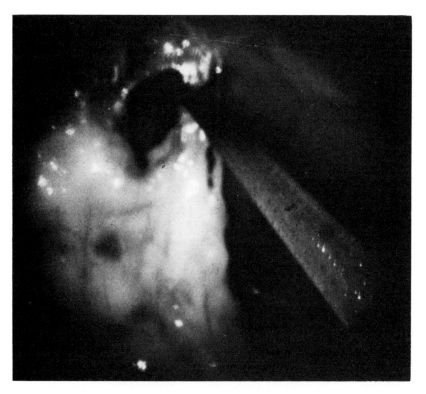

Fig. 9.15   Laparoscopic photograph of division of adhesions.

LAPAROSCOPIC EXAMINATION OF THE SMALL INTESTINE

External inspection

The small intestine can be examined at laparoscopy using the palpating probe or tubal grasping forceps introduced via an accessory trocar in the left hypochondrium. The procedure commences with the patient in the Trendelenberg position. Initially the caecum and appendix are located. The terminal ileum is picked up loop after loop and inspected. The inspected coils are then pushed to the upper abdomen. The procedure is continued until the whole of the ileum and lower jejunum has been inspected. Visualization of the upper jejunum is more difficult. The operating table is tilted 20° in a reversed Trendelenberg position. A second accessory trocar is introduced in the right hypochondrium along the linea semilunaris, through which is introduced a second palpating probe to lift the transverse colon and greater omentum. The first palpating probe is then used to inspect the upper jejunum starting from the duodenojejunal junction.

We have found laparoscopic inspection of the small bowel to be extremely useful and have been able to diagnose small bowel Crohn's disease and seromuscular tumours (leiomyomata and neurofibromata) which were missed by small bowel contrast studies. In addition the method can confirm small bowel kinking and dilatation in the blind loop syndrome as well as diagnosing Meckel's diverticulum and its complications. We have also encountered one instance of angiomatous malformation in a male patient with recurrent bleeding and negative angiography.

LAPAROSCOPIC HEPATIC LYMPHOGRAPHY

The technique of hepatic lymphography was pioneered by Müller and Meyer-Burg to study the lymphatic system of the liver in the normal state and in pathological conditions such as cirrhosis.[11–13] Subsequently the technique was extended to include the radiological visualization of the retrosternal lymph nodes.[14]

Lymphochromatography

The hepatic capsular lymphatics are easily outlined after the injection of Patent blue dye into the liver capsule. The dye is taken up and stains the lymph channels blue; they are then clearly visible through the laparoscopic telescope.

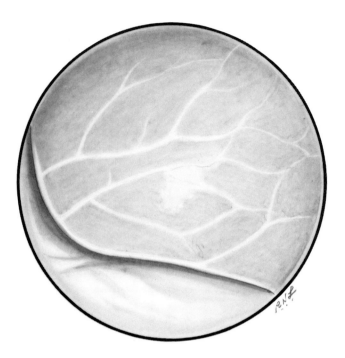

Fig. 9.16   The normal liver capsule has a fine network of lymph channels which appear as greyish-white delicate channels ramifying on top of the underlying hepatic parenchyma. The lymphatic network drains along collecting channels situated at the margin of the liver.

The normal capsular lymph vessels of the liver form a delicate network of fine greyish-white vessels throughout the surface of the hepatic lobes. This network drains into collecting vessels situated at the liver margin (Figure 9.16). The majority (80%) of hepatic lymph drains to the hilum of the liver and thence into the thoracic duct. However, lymph from the superior surface (approximately 20%) drains through lymph channels in the falciform ligament and diaphragm to the retrosternal lymph nodes and thence to the right lymphatic duct and to a lesser extent the thoracic duct (Figure 9.17). The two main abnormalities encountered in chronic liver disease are *capsular cloudiness* and *lymphectasia*. Capsular cloudiness results from the exudation of lymph protein due to an elevated endolymphatic pressure consequent on obstruction or excessive hepatic lymph production. The extravasated fibrinous exudate excites a fibrotic reaction in the liver capsule which assumes a frost-like cloudy appearance when seen through the laparoscope.

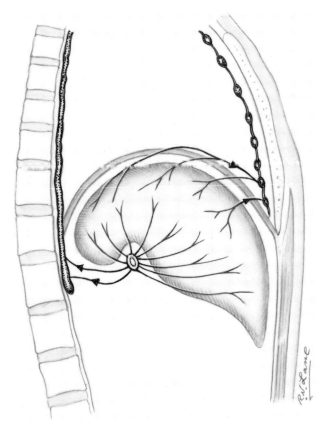

Fig. 9.17 Schematic representation of the lymph drainage of the liver. 80% of the lymph drains to the hilum of the liver and thence to the thoracic duct, but some lymph from the superior surface drains by lymph channels in the falciform ligament and diaphragm to the retrosternal nodes.

Lymphectasia is due to congestion of the surface lymphatics, which become enlarged and irregular and protrude beyond the liver surface. The dilated lymphatic channels have numerous constrictions which are caused by the valves within their lumen (Figure 9.18). Marked congestion and prominence of the capsular lymph vessels are commonly observed in chronic aggressive hepatitis and cirrhosis of the liver.

Retro-sternal lymphography

This procedure has been used in staging of patients with cancer of the breast and Hodgkin's disease. Following initial identification of the lymphatic channels in the falciform ligament by the injection of

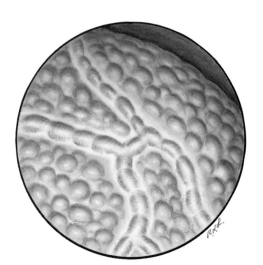

Fig. 9.18 Dilated prominent lymphatics are seen in chronic aggressive hepatitis and cirrhosis. The enlarged lymphatics have eccentric constrictions due to the lymph valves.

Patent blue in the liver capsule, a fine Chiba needle is guided percutaneously into a superficial lymph channel and oily contrast medium is injected. Both immediate and delayed films are taken. The technique outlines the retrosternal lymph node chain and the associated lymph channels.

REFERENCES

1   Royer, M., Mazuru, K. & Kohan, S. (1950) Biliary kinesia studied by means of peritoneoscopic cholangiography. *Gastroenterology, 16:* 83–90.
2   Berci, G., Morgenstern, L., Shore, J.M. & Shapiro, S. (1973) A direct approach to the differential diagnosis of jaundice. Laparoscopy with transhepatic cholecystocholangiography. *Am. J. Surg. 126:* 372–378.
3   Cuschieri, A. (1975) Value of laparoscopy in hepatobiliary disease. *Ann. R. Col. Surg. Eng. 57:* 33–38.
4   Irving, A.D. & Cuschieri, A. (1978) Laparoscopic assessment of the jaundiced patient. *Br. J. Surg. 65:* 678–680.
5   Meyer-Burg, J., Ziegler, U. & Palma, G. (1972) Zur supragastralen Pankreaskopie. Ergebnisse aus 125 Laparoskopien. *Dt. med. Wschr. 97:* 1969–1971.
6   Strauch, M., Lux, G. & Ottenjann, R. (1973) Infragastric pancreoscopy. *Endoscopy, 5:* 30–32.
7   Cuschieri, A., Hall, A.W. & Clark, J. (1978) Value of laparoscopy in the diagnosis and management of pancreatic carcinoma. *Gut, 19:* 672–677.
8   Allen, M.J., Borody, T.J., Bugliosi, T.F., May, G.R., LaRusso, N.F. & Johnson, L.T. (1985) Rapid dissolution of gallstones by methyl tert-butyl ether. Preliminary observations. *New Eng. J. Med., 312:* 217–220.
9   Sauerbruch, T., Deluis, M., Paumgartner, G., Holl, J., Wess, O., Wiber, W., Hepp, W. & Brendel, W. (1986) Fragmentation of gallstones by extracorporeal shock waves. *New Eng. J. Med. 314:* 818–820.

10   Wood, R.A.B. & Cuschieri, A. (1979) The patient with abdominal pain and negative investigations: discharge or laparoscopy. *Br. J. Surg. 66:* 900.

11   Meyer-Burg, J. (1972) The lymph system of the liver. I.Indirect visualization of the liver lymphatics with patent blue dye under peritoneoscopy. *Endoscopy (Stuttgart) 4:* 219–221.

12   Meyer-Burg, J. (1973) The lymphatic system of the liver. II. Direct laparoscopic observation of the lymphatic drainage with patent blue, [198]Au and lipiodol. *Endoscopy (Stuttgart) 5:* 32–35.

13   Müller, K. (1967) Laparoskopische Beobachtungen über den Lymphstrom der Leber. *Medsche Klin. 62:* 1500–1503.

14   Meyer-Burg, J., Schwoeror, I. & Arbieter, G. (1974) Die retrosternale Lymphografie. *Leber, Magen, Darm, 6:* 291–294.

10

Emergency Laparoscopy

ABDOMINAL TRAUMA

The introduction of abdominal lavage by Root and associates improved the diagnosis of intra-abdominal bleeding.[1] Subsequent experience with this test in patients with abdominal trauma has shown that not every haemoperitoneum requires exploration. Furthermore, the incidence of unnecessary diagnostic laparotomies in blunt abdominal trauma continues to average 20%. In a fifth of patients with a positive lavage subjected to laparotomy no visceral injury or continuing significant bleeding site is found at the time of surgery. Even the introduction of computed tomographic (CT) scanning has not eliminated the problem of unnecessary laparotomies in patients with trauma[2] and their consequences in terms of patient morbidity and hospital costs.

The idea of inspecting the abdominal cavity in emergency cases is not new.[3,4] Previous reports advocated the use of standard equipment, which though suitable for elective cases is not ideal for emergency work. For this reason we have developed a 4mm miniature laparoscope–the minilaparoscope–which approximates to the lavage catheter in diameter. It is easier, faster and safer to introduce than the larger instrument.[5] The examination can be performed in the emergency room, in the intensive care unit, on the stretcher or at the bedside, employing intravenous sedation and local anaesthesia.

In 1980 we reported our first results and updates of our clinical experience with minilaparoscopy were published later.[5,6,7]

Indications

Minilaparoscopy is particularly indicated in the following situations:

1 When the clinical picture and physical signs are obscured by an impaired level of consciousness induced by head injury, alcoholism, drug ingestion etc. such that it becomes impossible to reliably exclude intra-abdominal trauma on clinical grounds.

2 History or evidence of blunt abdominal trauma or abdominal stab wounds.

3 Unexplained hypotension.
4 Equivocal signs on physical examination in a conscious patient.

A rapid and accurate diagnostic technique allows proper assessment of the extent of injury and therefore the priorities of treatment, which can materially influence the eventual outcome of the severe trauma case. In our experience peritoneal lavage is unduly sensitive, and a positive result using the accepted criteria entails a laparotomy which is subsequently found to be unnecessary in 20% of patients, as the bleeding is observed to have stopped spontaneously by the time of surgery. The main value of minilaparoscopy is that it reliably indicates to the surgeon the need or otherwise for surgical intervention in trauma cases.

Technique

The complete set of instruments is assembled on a mobile trolley (Figures 10.1 and 10.2). The usual site of insertion for the pneumoperitoneum needle is immediately below the umbilicus in the midline. If previous abdominal scars are present, this site is changed to achieve the optimum intra-abdominal visualization. After local anaesthesia (1% lignocaine/lidocaine) and intravenous sedation with Diazemuls, a stab skin incision is made with a No. 11 blade to allow

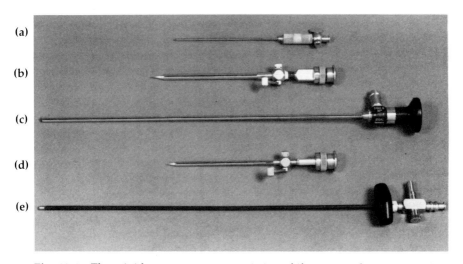

Fig. 10.1 The mini-laparoscope set, consisting of (from top to bottom) (a) pneumoperitoneum needle, (b) 5 mm examining trocar and cannula, (c) telescope (4 mm forward oblique), (d) second 4 mm accessory trocar, and (e) suction coagulation probe.

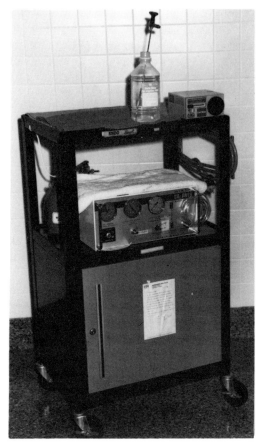

Fig. 10.2 The sterilized instruments and other accessories are kept in the bottom of this mobile trolley. On top is the attached examining light source and warm saline in a sterile plastic container. The telescope is immersed in this to avoid fogging after its introduction. The trolley, with the complete set of equipment can be moved to the emergency room or intensive care unit.

introduction of the spring-loaded pneumoperitoneum needle. When the peritoneal cavity has been entered, aspiration is performed to ensure that the needle has not penetrated a blood vessel or the lumen of the intestine. The needle is attached to an insufflation apparatus through which N_2O is delivered (rate: 1.0–1.2 l/min). For further technical details see Chapters 3–5. When an adequate pneumoperitoneum is achieved, the stab incision is slightly enlarged and the examining trocar (O.D. 5mm) is introduced through the previously established needle puncture site. The pre-warmed minilaparoscope is advanced through the examining trocar sheath.

Examination of the abdomen should be systematic, including all quadrants, the pelvis and the suprahepatic spaces. For the purposes of retraction, manipulation, suction or coagulation, a second, smaller, 4mm trocar and cannula may be introduced under direct vision, generally in the lateral right or left upper quadrant after injection of the lignocaine.

Following the examination, the abdomen is desufflated. The stab wounds are closed with one or two metallic clips. No antibiotics are administered unless there is an indication for antibiotic usage. The entire procedure should not exceed 15 to 20 minutes.

Haemoperitoneum

The pattern of distribution of blood can provide clues to the location of the bleeding site. A good example is seen with pelvic fractures, where the blood is mainly localized in the pelvic area. This is a major source for false-positive lavage results. The quantitative assessment of haemoperitoneum is difficult, but an impression can be gained with some experience and the following groups can be identified.

Minimal haemoperitoneum

A small amount of blood is seen in the lateral peritoneal gutter or streaks of blood are discovered between intestinal loops. If this small volume remains unchanged and the search for the bleeding site has been negative, the patient can be observed. If the bleeding site is found, it may be seen to be oozing minimally or to have stopped. In our series of this type of patient the bleeding site was discovered in only half. Extremely small volumes of blood in the peritoneal cavity can be sufficient to provide a positive lavage.

Moderate haemoperitoneum

Obvious blood pooling (5–10 mm deep) is observed in the paracolic gutters. In this situation the second accessory trocar is introduced under visual control after infiltration with local anaesthetic, and the suction cannula is advanced. The haemoperitoneum is evacuated and a systematic search for the injury is initiated. The suction cannula itself is used as a palpating probe. It is used gently to elevate omentum, intestinal loops etc. If a bleeding site is found, for example a lacerated liver, the injury is watched through the laparoscope. If the bleeding is brisk, surgical intervention is indicated. If the bleeding site is not discovered after 5 to 10 minutes of diligent search, but the paracolic gutters refill with blood to the previous level, the bleeding vessel is probably not within the range of visualization, and surgical intervention is necessary. A small oozing laceration which shows signs of spontaneous haemostasis or lesions with an adherent blood clot without bleeding can be managed conservatively. In patients with moderate haemoperitoneum laparoscopy allows the surgeon to formulate a safe management policy.

If injuries are found which require immediate operation, precise location of the injury to a particular quadrant facilitates selection of the optimal incision. The suction–coagulation probe may be applied in assessing oozing lesions, or in selected cases aimed coagulation can be applied *provided CO_2 and not N_2O has been used for the peritoneal insufflation.*

Severe haemoperitoneum

If the initial pneumoperitoneum needle aspiration yields blood in the syringe on two or three attempts or subsequent to insufflation, the laparoscopic view displays intestinal loops floating in, or surrounded by, a pool of blood the indication for immediate operation is obvious. In these patients, two or more fingerbreadths of blood are present in the paracolic gutters.

Organ perforations

In patients who sustain hollow visceral injury, yellowish fluid is observed in the paracolic gutters. The fluid should be aspirated and sent for analysis (amylase, bile, pH, culture, etc.), but in general this finding is an indication for surgery. If several hours have elapsed between the trauma and admission, the injury may not be seen, but it may be suspected by indirect findings such as an omental mass in one particular region, or adherent oedematous, hyperaemic intestinal loops. The palpation probe can be of help by moving these loops or the omentum. However, perforation of the retroperitoneal segment of the duodenum – the third part – and pancreatic injuries cannot be visualized. Fortunately, these lesions are rare and other diagnostic measures will help to clarify the clinical picture.

Splenic injuries

There are characterized by accumulation of blood in the left paracolic gutter. The omentum covering the spleen is elevated by a pool of blood or a blood clot presenting as a bluish-tinted elevated omentum is seen in this area. Splenic conservation in suitable cases is a desirable objective.[8] In some cases, the laparoscope reveals only minimal haemoperitoneum in this area, without significant bulging or bluish discolouration of the covering omentum. Even if the spleen scan denotes injury, if vital signs are stable the patient can be managed nonoperatively with very careful observation. A normal size spleen is usually not seen in the left upper gutter because it is covered by omentum.

Liver injuries

Deceleration injuries are frequently characterized by lacerations on the anterior surface or dome of the liver lobes and on the round or falciform ligament. These lacerations can be clearly seen using the laparoscope. The undersurface can be inspected with a palpation probe which can gently lift up segments of the right lobe and the entire left lobe. If lacerations are discovered, the telescope is advanced and close observation under magnification is performed for a few minutes. In case of a small oozing laceration, compression or coagulation may be used. If after a prolonged period of observation bleeding persists laparotomy must be considered.

Penetrating injuries

We do not laparoscope patients who sustain gunshot wounds. However, penetrating stab wounds are an indication for laparoscopy. In a recent review of 89 cases of stab wounds of the abdomen, there had been unnecessary exploration in one-third.[9] Our approach to these cases is as follows: the skin wound is temporarily closed to provide a seal for the pneumoperitoneum. The penetration of the parietal peritoneum can be either excluded or confirmed with great certainty. If there has been penetration, the underlying area is inspected using the palpation probe, lifting up the loops of intestine to check for bleeding points, serosal injuries, leakage or other signs of perforation.

Results in 129 cases

Negative laparoscopy – no exploration

In 72 cases (55.8%) no haemoperitoneum or other abnormality was discovered. None of these patients subsequently required an exploratory laparotomy.

Positive laparoscopy – no exploration

In 33 patients (25.5%) minimal to moderate haemoperitoneum was found, but no identifiable injury or only minimal lacerations could be discovered. These patients were observed in the intensive care unit. Only one of this group required laparotomy.

A 35-year-old white male was admitted after a motor vehicle accident with a compression skull fracture in a semi-comatose state. Laparoscopy revealed minimal haemoperitoneum in the left lower paracolic gutter without other abnormalities. The patient's condition improved and he was started on oral feeding on the third postadmission day. Some days later the patient developed left lower quadrant pain, with fever and leukocytosis and he was explored on the eighth day. A sealed perforation of the sigmoid colon near the recto-sigmoid junction was found. In retrospect, the minimal haemoperitoneum in the left lower quadrant and the persistent pneumoperitoneum should have been an indication for a contrast enema at an earlier stage.

Positive laparoscopy – exploration

In 24 patients (18.6%) severe haemoperitoneum was discovered. The laparoscopic findings were confirmed at surgery. In all but one patient the source of bleeding or organ perforation was located: in this one exception 700 ml of blood was evacuated at operation but no bleeding source found. The 24 cases included 3 liver lacerations, 11 splenic injuries (in 6 patients the spleen was conserved with splenorrhaphy), 4 organ perforations and 6 arterial bleeding points.

Complications

In one patient a minimal amount of haemoperitoneum was interpreted as being due to injury to the omentum during the trocar insertion. Fresh coagulum was seen around the area. The patient was kept under observation and made an uneventful recovery.

ACUTE ABDOMEN

In the vast majority of cases the diagnosis of the common intra-abdominal emergencies is made on clinical assessment and routine biochemical tests, radiology and ultrasound scanning. Nevertheless, problems are encountered from time to time regarding both the exact diagnosis and the need for surgical intervention. In these situations minilaparoscopy may provide useful information which materially influences management. The technique is particularly useful in the following situations.

Female patients with acute onset right iliac fossa pain where the differentiation between acute appendicitis, ectopic pregnancy and bacterial salpingitis is difficult. The diagnosis can be firmly and rapidly established by laparoscopy and those patients with salpingitis can be spared unnecessary surgical intervention. Culture material can be obtained through the suction cannula for bacterial analysis and antibiotic therapy started.

Suspected mesenteric ischaemia. In the absence of the full-blown clinical picture, the diagnosis of mesenteric vascular insufficiency can be difficult and there is no reliable diagnostic test. Often these patients are old and have coexistent cardiovascular and respiratory disease which renders them poor operative risks. Laparoscopy is eminently suitable for the detection of ischaemic bowel and for establishing the need for active intervention. In these patients we prefer to perform the procedure under general endotracheal anaesthesia in the operating theatre and proceed immediately to laparotomy if the diagnosis is confirmed. It is therefore essential that consent be obtained for laparotomy in addition to laparoscopy before the patient is anaesthetized.

Visualization of the small bowel and colon is greatly facilitated during laparoscopy by the use of a secondary trocar in the left upper quadrant along the lateral margin of the rectus muscle for insertion of the palpating probe. However, great care must be observed in lifting ischaemic bowel loops since the risk of perforation by the palpating probe is high. The loops should be gently teased by the probe rather than lifted and diagnosis based on dusky appearance, lack of serosal sheen and absence of peristalsis when the bowel is touched with the palpating probe. The procedure has also been used instead of second-look laparotomy in those patients in whom bowel of questionable viability was left at the time of the initial surgical intervention. Again, the second-look minilaparoscopy is performed under general anaesthesia in these patients.

Acute upper abdominal pain. Although differentiation between perforated peptic ulcer and acute cholecystitis or pancreatitis is usually obvious from clinical examination, laboratory results and plain erect and supine radiographs of the abdomen, diagnostic difficulties may be encountered. In practice, the important differentiation is that between acute perforation without obvious subphrenic gas and acute pancreatitis, especially when the serum amylase is only moderately elevated. This dilemma is easily solved by minilaparoscopy, the findings of which will indicate whether there is a need for operative intervention.

REFERENCES

1   Root, H.O., Hauser, C.W., McKinley, C.R., LaFave, J.W. & Mendiola, R.P. (1965) Diagnostic peritoneal lavage. *Surgery, 57:* 633–637.
2   Federle, M.P., Crass, A., Brooke, J. & Trunkey, D.O. (1982) Computed tomography in blunt abdominal trauma. *Archs Surg. 117:* 645–650.
3   Gazzaniga, A.B., Slanton, W.W. & Bartlett, R.H. (1976) Laparoscopy in the diagnosis of blunt and penetrating injuries to the abdomen. *Am. J. Surg. 131:* 315–318.
4   Carnevale, N., Baron, N. & Delany, H.M. (1977) Peritoneoscopy as an aid in the diagnosis of abdominal trauma: a preliminary report. *J. Trauma, 17:* 634–641.
5   Sherwood, R., Berci, G., Austin, E. & Morgenstern, L. (1980) Minilaparoscopy for blunt abdominal trauma. *Archs Surg. 115:* 672–673.
6   Berci, G., Dunkelman, D., Michel, S.L., Sanders, G., Wahlstrom, E. & Morgenstern, L. (1983) Emergency minilaparoscopy in abdominal trauma. An update. *Am. J. Surg. 146:* 261–265.
7   Berci, G. & Wahlstrom, E. (1985) Emergency laparoscopy. In *Surgical Endoscopy.* Dent, L. (ed.) pp. 478–483. Chicago: Year Book Medical Publishers.
8   Morgenstern, L. & Shapiro, S.J. (1979) Techniques of splenic conservation. *Archs Surg. 114:* 449–454.
9   Donaldson, L.A., Findlay, I.G. & Smith, A. (1981) A retrospective review of 89 stab wounds to the abdomen. *Br. J. Surg. 68:* 793–796.

11
Laparoscopy for Abdominal Malignancy

There is little doubt that laparoscopy has been grossly under-utilized in the management of patients with cancer, although there has been an increased use reported in patients with abdominal malignancy in recent years.[1-5] The main reasons are the ready availability of non-invasive investigations such as CT scanning and the general lack of training in laparoscopy, which means that only a small percentage of practising surgeons and gastroenterologists are familiar with the technique. Yet the advantages to the patients and the savings to any health care system which emanate from the routine or selective use of laparoscopy are considerable. This is an investigation which is cheap, reliable, obtains tissue for diagnosis and can avoid the use of expensive investigations. It can and often does spare patients from unwarranted surgical intervention for advanced non-resectable malignancy and thus spares these unfortunate patients needless pain and anxiety in addition to reducing time spent in hospital. Less frequently, but by no means rarely, a laparoscopic examination will indicate that a patient previously assessed as having advanced incurable malignant disease in fact has resectable and potentially curable cancer. Several such instances have been encountered by the authors during the last 15 years. For example, a 50-year-old female with a carcinoma of the breast, multiple hepatic filling defects in her isotope liver scan and a raised alkaline phosphatase activity, was shown by laparoscopy to have a previously undiagnosed polycystic liver.

There have been a number of studies which have compared the diagnostic yield of laparoscopy with those of isotope scintiscanning and ultrasound examination of the liver in the detection of hepatic secondaries.[6-9] These have consistently shown that laparoscopy is superior to these diagnostic modalities in terms of its overall diagnostic rate, sensitivity and specificity.

INDICATIONS

For logistic reasons laparoscopy cannot be used in all patients with cancer. The procedure is likely to impart useful information in the following:

131

1 Patients suspected of having primary hepatobiliary cancer.
2 Patients with a diagnosis of pancreatic cancer.
3 Patients with ascites thought to be caused by peritoneal dissemination.
4 Patients with breast, bronchial, oesophageal and gastro-intestinal cancer who have abnormal liver function tests or in whom preoperative assessment suggests advanced, inoperable or metastatic disease.
5 Some patients with Hodgkin's or non-Hodgkin's lymphoma.
6 Suspicion of intra-abdominal cancer.
7 Second-look assessment.

LIVER TUMOURS

Benign tumours

The benign lesions which can be visualized by laparoscopy are adenoma, primary and secondary haemangioma and solitary or multiple microhamartoma (cholangioma, von Meyenburg's complex).

Adenoma

This appears as a greyish-white smooth swelling with a fine meshwork of surface vessels. The liver parenchyma around its base extends as a thin layer for a few millimetres along the sides of the swelling. The adenoma feels firm to hard on palpation with the probe. The lesion is usually solitary and like focal nodular hyperplasia is encountered with increased frequency in females on oral contraception.[10] Biopsy is best performed with the fine-pointed biopsy (Robbers) forceps. Resolution of hepatic adenoma after cessation of oral contraceptives is best documented by follow-up laparoscopy which is essential if a decision is made not to intervene surgically in the first instance.

Haemangiomas

These vascular malformations are classified as primary when they are observed in an otherwise normal liver and secondary when they arise within a chronically diseased liver (post-necrotic scarring, chronic aggressive hepatitis and cirrhosis). Most are cavernous haemangiomas and appear as multiloculated, dark-blue elevated surface lesions. They are easily compressible with the palpating probe and refill immediately on release of pressure. They vary considerably in size and in extreme cases may extend over most of one lobe. *Haemangiomas must never be biopsied*, as this is invariably followed by torrential haemorrhage. If large or in any way contributing to the patient's symptoms, the safest policy is surgical excision.

Microhamartomas

These may be solitary or multiple and generalized and are seen as granular whitish nodules on the liver surface. Laparoscopically they cannot be distinguished from other miliary foci such as tuberculosis, sarcoidosis and secondary deposits. For this reason, multiple biopsies are necessary. Histologically they appear as well encapsulated cystic cholangiomata with ductal plate malformation and chronic inflammatory cell infiltrate. They are generally regarded as congenital developmental anomalies. However, similar lesions have been produced in animals following administration of carcinogenic compounds and exposure to irradiation.

Hepatocellular carcinoma

The laparoscopic appearances differ depending on whether the tumour arises in an otherwise normal hepatic parenchyma or in a cirrhotic liver.[11-13] Clinically the onset of a hepatocellular carcinoma in patients with chronic liver disease is marked by a rapid deterioration in their general condition.

Cirrhomimetic hepatocellular carcinoma

It can be very difficult to detect a carcinoma in an end-stage cirrhotic liver. When evident, the tumour, which is often multicentric, appears as areas of white nodular tissue in between the regenerating nodules or in the septal scars. Large obvious tumour masses are seldom encountered. Multiple biopsies of the suspicious areas are essential. Not infrequently, however, despite an elevated α-fetoprotein and a marked deterioration in the patient's general condition, the laparoscopic macroscopic appearances are simply those of an advanced disordered cirrhosis.

Hepatocellular carcinoma in a normal liver

This has a distinctive appearance which usually, but not always, allows differentiation from secondary hepatic tumour deposits. In the first place a hepatocellular carcinoma never erupts through the liver

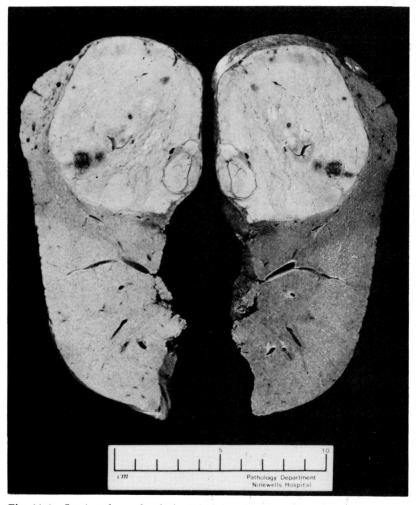

Fig. 11.1 Section through whole right lobe of liver containing a hepatoma stained for iron. The tumour appears white in contrast to the dark staining liver parenchyma. This difference is due to the inability of the hepatoma cells to store iron.

parenchyma and does not become umbilicated. Instead it presents as a pale smooth elevation with thinned out hepatic capsule and superficial parenchyma. Often the related Glisson's capsule has large tortuous veins draining the tumour. The reason for the pale appearance in contrast to the darker normal hepatic parenchyma is that hepatic carcinoma cells are unable to store iron. This is well demonstrated in Figure 11.1, which is a resected specimen of a right lobe hepatoma stained for iron with Perl's Prussian Blue. Primary hepatocellular carcinoma is best biopsied by a long-shaft Menghini or Tru-cut needle introduced at the centre of the protuberant area and avoiding any large surface vessels, which if traumatized can bleed profusely. Surface brush biopsy of the lesions is a useful technique for obtaining a definitive cytological diagnosis.

Aside from outlining the diagnosis, laparoscopy can be extremely useful in assessing the operability of these neoplasms and also to ascertain the extent of liver resection necessary for complete and intact removal of the tumour

Secondary hepatic deposits

The detection of secondary tumour deposits in the liver together with a target biopsy under vision, which allows histological confirmation of the diagnosis and the tumour type is one of the most important uses of laparoscopy.[15] The practical benefits in terms of patient care and avoidance of needless expensive investigations and surgical intervention are obvious. On the other hand, the demonstration of a more favourable tumour deposit such as carcinoid may indicate a more aggressive approach with palliative resection and intra-arterial hepatic chemofusor therapy.

In terms of their laparoscopic appearances secondary deposits in the liver may be described as discretely nodular, expansive nodular, nodular infiltrating, miliary and diffusely infiltrating (Figure 11.2).

Discretely nodular

These appear as creamy white surface tumour nodules erupting through the liver surface with intervening normal parenchyma (see Colour Plates 7 and 8). As a result of central necrosis and fibrosis, some but not all of these tumour nodules are umbilicated. Others may be surrounded by a zone of venous congestion which appears as a bluish rim extending some 1–2 cm around the lesions. This change is most commonly seen in deposits from bronchial carcinoma. It is different from peliosis hepatis which may also be encountered in secondary hepatic tumours. Nodular discrete metastases appear particularly striking in the presence of malignant bile duct obstruction as the whitish tumour deposits contrast strikingly with the dark green hepatic parenchyma. Metastases from malignant melanoma are often heavily pigmented and therefore appear darker than the surrounding hepatic parenchyma.

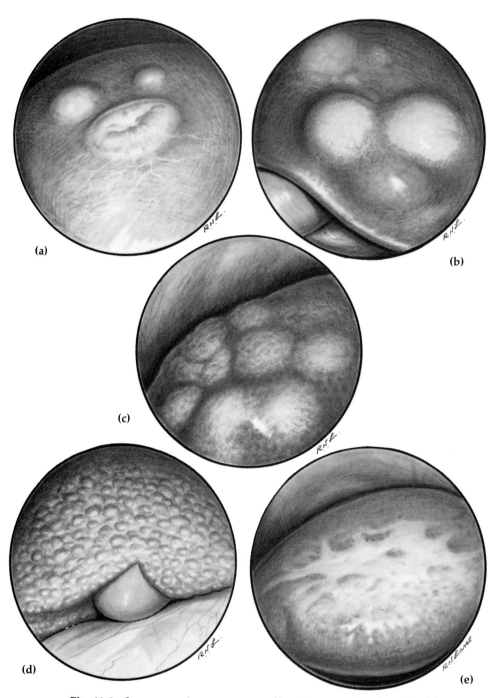

Fig. 11.2 Laparoscopic appearances of hepatic secondary deposits: (a) discretely nodular; (b) nodular expansive; (c) nodular infiltrating; (d) miliary; (e) diffuse infiltrating.

Nodular expansive

These comprise large well defined solitary or multiple tumour masses. On target biopsy with the Menghini needle some of these masses are found to be cystic due to central liquefactive necrosis. The tumours which commonly give rise to nodular expansive deposits include carcinoid, colorectal adenocarcinoma, thyroid carcinoma and malignant islet cell tumours.

Nodular infiltrating

Large areas of the liver are seen through the laparoscope to be replaced by confluent nodular tumour masses which appear to have coalesced from initial growth as separate nodules. These appearances are usually encountered in highly malignant anaplastic lesions, such as round cell carcinoma of the bronchus and indicate a poor prognosis, with very limited survival.

Miliary

The liver surface is seen through the laparoscope to be studded by small white yellowish white nodules, the appearances of which are non-specific and cannot be differentiated from other miliary foci such as tuberculosis and sarcoidosis. Miliary metastases are often seen in patients with lymphomas although they can be encountered in a variety of carcinomas.

Diffuse infiltrating

Large areas of the liver are entirely replaced by creamy white tumour tissue without the formation of nodules. The liver is rigid on palpation, with rounded anterior margins. Often it is difficult to recognize any normal hepatic parenchyma. This type of secondary tumour deposit is rapidly lethal and all of the 52 patients in the author's series were dead within six weeks of laparoscopic diagnosis. These patients are usually terminal and should be spared any active therapy except pain relief and sedation.

*Effect of laparoscopic assessment of hepatic tumour deposits
on patient management*

Apart from obtaining histological confirmation of the diagnosis, the laparoscopic appearances influence the management of the individual patient and laparoscopy can be extremely useful in this respect.

In the first instance, the documentation of extensive hepatic involvement should indicate to the sensible clinician that the time to call off any active treatment has been reached and terminal nursing care with adequate pain relief and sedation is the only sensible option.

There has been a resurgence of hepatic resection for a solitary metastasis particularly when due to colorectal cancer. Reliance on assessment by investigative modalities such as hepatic scanning with CT, scintigraphy and ultrasound may lead to errors in selection of patients for surgery and it is the author's practice to laparoscope all these patients prior to surgical intervention. Not infrequently the 'solitary metastasis' is observed to be multiple at laparoscopy, with one large deposit and several surface miliary lesions in both lobes.

Finally, new chemotherapeutic approaches for hepatic secondary deposits are being used and assessed in both retrospective and prospective trials. A prior assessment of the true extent of hepatic involvement is necessary but has been consistently overlooked in many of these studies. This is very important as the survival of the untreated patient with hepatic deposits depends largely on the pattern and extent of liver involvement by the metastatic tumour.

The laparoscopic appearances of carcinoma of the gallbladder are discussed in Chapter 8 and the approach to examination of pancreatic swellings and carcinoma is outlined in Chapter 9.

LAPAROSCOPY FOR GASTROINTESTINAL CANCER

Several reported series have demonstrated the value of staging laparoscopy prior to surgical intervention for oesophageal carcinoma.[9,16,17] In the Russian study 16 out of 65 patients (23%) were found by laparoscopy to have extensive abdominal spread of the disease.[17] In a recent British study laparoscopy was found to be superior to hepatic scintigraphy and ultrasound examination in the detection of secondary deposits from gastric and oesophageal cancer.[9] The procedure was also found to be helpful in obviating the need for laparotomy in oesophageal cancer. These authors concluded that whilst laparoscopy should be used routinely as preoperative staging in patients with oesophageal cancer, its value in gastric cancer is doubtful as a high proportion of patients require at least palliative surgery. This latter statement does not accord with our experience[14] and that reported by others.[18–20] In the Manchester study 17 out of 25 patients with gastric cancer were considered to be inoperable and only 5 of the inoperable patients subsequently required palliative surgical intervention; these five included three who had endoscopic oesophageal intubation for dysphagia.[20] In our experience with preoperative staging for gastric carcinoma by laparoscopy, the extent of local invasion of the adjacent organs by the gastric carcinoma tends to be underestimated. Thus some cases judged to be operable by laparoscopy are subsequently found to be non-resectable at laparotomy.

Rectal carcinoma, especially of the upper and middle third, is eminently suitable for preoperative assessment by laparoscopy. It is therefore surprising that there have been few reports on its use in these patients. The results of one published report[21] clearly indicates the usefulness of the procedure in outlining advanced disease which precludes attempts at excisional surgery.

The question which has to be addressed is whether laparoscopy should be used routinely or selectively in oesophageal, gastric and rectal cancer. After a decade of its use, our opinion has changed towards the latter option since routine laparoscopy in all these patients imposes an inordinate case load. Laparoscopy should therefore be used when the preoperative tests, clinical features and assessment indicate a strong possibility of advanced or metastatic disease. This selective use is certainly worth while and constitutes our current practice.

LAPAROSCOPY FOR HODGKIN'S DISEASE

Staging laparotomy for Hodgkin's disease is on the decline and is nowadays largely restricted to clinical stage I and II patients. Several reports in recent years have indicated that laparoscopy with hepatic and splenic biopsy may be a viable and safer alternative at least in some patients.[22-26] However, the exact role of this investigation is yet to be defined and to date it does not appear to be used routinely in the management of these patients except in a few centres.

There is undoubted evidence that laparoscopy can rapidly confirm clinical stage III and IV disease and allow histological confirmation and typing in these patients.[22,23] In patients with suspected clinical stage I and II, there is good evidence that laparoscopy with liver and splenic biopsy may obviate the necessity for staging laparotomy in up to 70% of patients.[24,25]

Laparoscopic staging for Hodgkin's disease should always be done in an operating theatre under general anaesthesia with cross-matched blood being readily available. The reasons for this are twofold. First, it is essential that the liver and spleen can be seen adequately, and this requires paralysed abdominal musculature and facilities for adequate positional change. Secondly, biopsy of the spleen is often necessary. This procedure is always followed by haemorrhage, which usually stops spontaneously but often requires volume replacement using colloids or blood transfusion. In addition 3–5% require surgical intervention for continued bleeding, when splenectomy should be performed.

Staging laparoscopy for Hodgkin's disease also necessitates routine liver biopsy. If obvious hepatic lesions are seen these are biopsied under vision. Often non-specific mesenchymal reactions of the liver such as exaggeration of the lobular pattern, thickening of the capsule and congested surface lymph vessels are seen without any obvious hepatic involvement by the neoplastic process. In these instances several Tru-cut or Menghini needle biopsies are taken from both lobes. The macroscopic appearances of liver involvement by Hodgkin's disease have been classified by Beck into miliary, conglomerate, nodular and diffuse.[27] The conglomerate and nodular forms are best biopsied by Robbers forceps, the miliary and diffuse varieties by the needle-core technique. Again, several biopsies should be taken.

Whether enlarged or not, the spleen must be adequately visualized by positioning the table in the reversed Trendelenberg position with rotation to the right. Any residual covering omentum is gently teased away with the palpating probe. Exophytic lesions are best biopsied using fine-pointed Robbers biopsy forceps. Otherwise a fine-needle core biopsy is taken. The incidence of severe and continued bleeding is very high in patients with very large and congested spleens; needle biopsy is best avoided in these patients.

REFERENCES

1 Sugarbaker, P.H. & Wilson, R.E. (1976) Using celioscopy to determine stages of intra-abdominal neoplasms. *Archs Surg. 111:* 41–44.
2 Ozols, R.F., Fisher, R.I., Anderson, T. et al. (1981) Peritoneoscopy in the management of ovarian cancer. *Am. J. Obstet. Gynec. 140:* 611–619.
3 Bleiberg, H., Rozencweig, M., Mathieu, M. et al. (1978) The use of peritoneoscopy in the detection of liver metastases. *Cancer, 41:* 863–867.
4 Cuschieri, A., Hall, A.W. & Clark, J. (1978) Value of laparoscopy in the diagnosis and management of pancreatic carcinoma. *Gut, 19:* 672–677.
5 Hall, T.J., Donaldson, D.R. & Brennan, R.H. (1980) Laparoscopy under local anaesthesia in 250 medical and surgical patients. *Br. J. Surg. 67:* 751–753.
6 Canossi, G.C., Cortesi, N., Manenti, A. & Givertini, Jr, G. (1975) Scintigrafia epatica e laparoscopica nella ricerca della metastasi del fegato: osservazioni comparative in 112 casi. *Minerva Chir. 30:* 126–130.

7   Margolis, R., Hansen, H.H., Muggia, F.M. & Kanhouwa, S. (1974) Diagnosis of liver metastases in bronchogenic carcinoma. A comparative study of liver scans, function tests and peritoneoscopy with liver biopsy in 111 patients. *Cancer (Philadelphia), 34:* 1825–1829.

8   Sauer, R., Fahrländer, H. & Friedrich, R. (1973) Comparison of the accuracy of liver scans and peritoneoscopy in benign and malignant primary and metastatic tumours of the liver. 222 confirmed cases examined by both methods simultaneously. *Scand. J. Gastroenterol. 8:* 389–394.

9   Shandall, A. & Johnson, C. (1985) Laparoscopy or scanning in oesophageal and gastric carcinoma? *Br. J. Surg. 22:* 449–451.

10 Kinch, R. & Lough, J. (1978) Focal nodular hyperplasia of the liver and oral contraceptives. *Am. J. Obstet. Gynec. 132:* 717.

11 Etienne, J.P., Chaput, J.C., Feydy, P. & Gueroult, N. (1973) La laparoscopie dans le cancer primitif du foie de l'adulte. *Ann. Gastroenterol. Hepatol. 9:* 49–56.

12 Pergola, F., Lignereux, J. & Cachin, M. (1961) Les aspects laparoscopiques du cancer primitif du foie. *Sem. Hôp. Paris, 37:* 2433–2435.

13 Delavierre, P. & Martignon, C. (1975) La biopsie et la cytologie laparoscopiques dans les cancers primitifs et secondaires du foie. *Ann. Gastroenterol. Hepatol. 11:* 475.

14 Cuschieri, A. (1980) Laparoscopy in general surgery and gastroenterology. *Br. J. Hosp. Med. 24:* 252–258.

15 Jori, G.P. & Peschle, C. (1972) Combined peritoneoscopy and liver biopsy in the diagnosis of hepatic neoplasm. *Gastroenterology, 62:* 1016–1019.

16 Grosse, H.J. & Müller, K. (1971) Kombinierte Gastro-Ösophago-Laparoskopie. *Dtsch. Med. 22:* 364–366.

17 Sotnikou, V.N., Ermolov, A.S., Litvinov, S.S. et al. (1973) Diagnostika Vnutriabdominalnykh metastazov raka pishchevoda putem laparoskopii (diagnoses of intra-abdominal metastases of esophageal cancer by laparoscopy). *Vop. Onkol. 19:* 35–38.

18 Berezov, I.U.E., Sotnikov, V.N. & Lapin, M.D. (1972) Vozmozhnosti laparoskopii prirake zheludka (laparoscopy in gastric cancer). *Vop. Onkol. 18:* 26–31.

19 Nikora, P.I. (1971) Laparoskopiia pri rake proksimalnogo otdela zheludka (laparoscopy in cancer of the proximal region of the stomach). *Vop. Onkol. 17:* 85–90.

20 Gross, E., Bancewicz, J. & Ingram, G. (1984) Assessment of gastric carcinoma by laparoscopy. *Br. med. J. 288:* 157.

21 Atanov, I.U.P. & Gallinger, I.U.I. (1972) Laparoskopiia v diagnostike nekotorykh opukhole i bruishno i polosti (laparoscopy in the diagnosis of several abdominal tumours). *Sov. Med. 35:* 93–98.

22 Devita, V.T., Bagley, Jr, C.H., Goodell, B. et al. (1971) Peritoneoscopy in the staging of Hodgkin's disease. *Cancer Res. 31:* 1746–1750.

23 Bagley Jr, C.M., Roth, J.A., Thomas, L.B. & Devita, V.T. (1972) Liver biopsy in Hodgkin's disease. Clinicopathologic correlations in 127 patients. *Ann. intern. Med. 76:* 219–225.

24 Coleman, M., Lightdale, C.J., Vinceguerra, V.P. et al. (1976) Peritoneoscopy in Hodgkin's disease: confirmation of results by laparotomy. *J. Am. med. Ass. 236:* 2634–2636.

25 Spinelli, P., Beretta, G., Bayetta, E. et al. (1975) Laparoscopy and

laparotomy combined with bone marrow biopsy in staging of Hodgkin's disease. *Br. med. J. iv:* 554–556.

26   Veronesi, U., Spinelli, P., Bonadonna, G. et al. (1976) Laparoscopy and laparotomy in staging Hodgkin's and non-Hodgkin's lymphoma. *Am. J. Roentg. 127:* 501–503.

27   Beck, K. (1984) *Colour Atlas of Laparoscopy* p. 276. Philadelphia: Saunders.

28   Berci, G., Shore, J.M., Panish, J. & Morgenstern, L. (1973) The evaluation of a new peritoneoscope as a diagnostic aid to the surgeon. *Ann. Surg. 178:* 37–44.

29   McCallum, R.W. & Berci, G. (1976) Laparoscopy in hepatic disease. *Gastrointest. Endosc. 23:* 20–24.

12
Gynaecological Laparoscopy

Geoffrey Chamberlain

Viewing the peritoneal cavity through a laparoscope has been done for eighty years. Many surgeons and gynaecologists in the early years of this century performed the operation, which they variously called peritoneoscopy, pelviscopy, coelioscopy or laparoscopy; of these the last name is now the most widely used.[1] However, the wider use of the technique has followed the invention of fibre-optic conducted light and improved lens systems.

SPECIAL INSTRUMENTS FOR GYNAECOLOGICAL LAPAROSCOPY

Two major varieties of laparoscope are used in gynaecology:

1 A simple diagnostic light transmission and lens system (Figure 12.1b). For any procedure in the pelvic cavity, a double puncture must be performed so that all ancillary instruments can be manipulated through a separate small trocar passed through the second incision.

2 An operating laparoscope, which has a built-in operating channel through which ancillary instruments can be inserted. The eyepiece is offset to the side of the instrument to allow this and two prisms are introduced in the optical system (Figure 12.1b).

The simple diagnostic laparoscope can obviously be thinner (4–6mm diameter) than the operating variety (10–12mm diameter). The operating instrument requires only one abdominal incision, but the surgeon must become accustomed to a slight loss in light intensity and clarity due to the prism systems; further, the operating instruments can encroach upon the field of vision and some gynaecologists find it difficult to judge the depth of the operating field visually.

Trocars and cannulas are made with an internal diameter which allows an air-tight fit but usually permits easy passage of the accompanying laparoscope. The faceted-point trocar is easier to insert

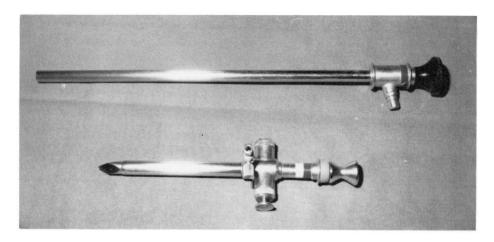

(a)

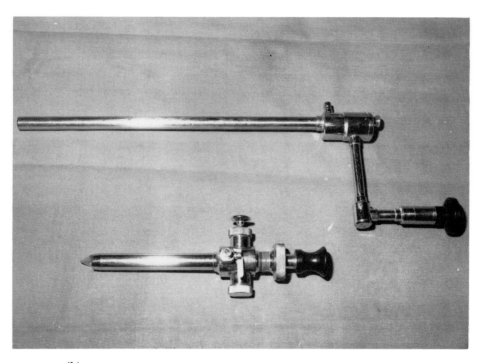

(b)

Fig. 12.1   (a) A diagnostic laparoscope and trocar; (b) an operating
laparoscope and trocar.

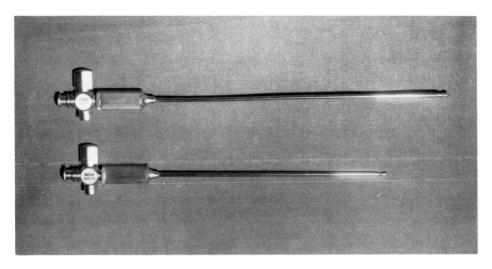

Fig. 12.2   Veress needles for insufflation.

through the abdominal wall than the conical point trocar. The linea alba should be pierced just inferior to the umbilicus. Insulated cannulae are safer if electrocautery is to be used in case there is an accidental contact between the electric equipment inside the pelvic cavity and the tip of the cannula. The cannulae need careful handling when being washed, dried or during sterilization, since knocks can distort their internal diameter.

The cold light source can be either one of the cheaper tungsten halogen systems or the more powerful but expensive xenon light source. The latter is essential if photography or television viewing are contemplated. The light is conveyed through a fibre-optic cable, which must fit well with both the projector at one end and the telescope at the other; light is lost with badly fitting connectors, especially if there are gaps at the connection points. The numerous glass fibres in the bundle can be damaged by acute bending of the cable or by dropping the instrument. Some light transmission cables are fluid-filled and are therefore more robust, but these cannot be sterilized by gas or autoclaving.

Gas insufflation is initiated by inserting a Veress pneumoperitoneum needle (Figure 12.2). A spring-loaded blunt end extends beyond the sharp point of the cannula to allow safer intraperitoneal manoeuvring. The needles can be obtained from 8 cm to 15 cm in length; the longer ones are essential for operating on obese patients since the gynaecologist approaches the peritoneal cavity obliquely.

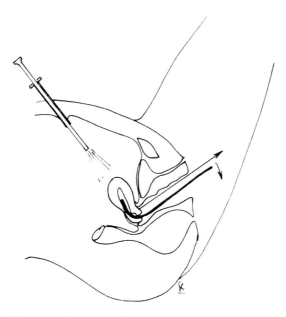

Fig. 12.3 Diagram of the uterine manipulation required to provide vision to all parts of the pelvis at laparoscopy.

Every operating theatre where laparoscopy is performed must have a supply of the longer needles.

Uterine manipulation through the vagina is required to allow the operator to view all parts of the pelvis (Figure 12.3). In most instances, a Hegar dilator within the cavity with a vulsellum forceps on the anterior lip of the cervix allows adequate control and facilitates manoeuvring the uterus through its full range. If a dye insufflation is indicated, a hollow cannula with a rubber or metal occluding acorn will be needed.

Many other instruments are available for laparoscopy. The range of biopsy forceps, probes and scissors is wide and minor variations must be assessed. The gynaecologist should borrow samples for trial before purchasing the equipment. In the UK the Royal College of Obstetricians and Gynaecologists will provide members with a useful booklet about the relative merits of all laparoscopy equipment available in the United Kingdom.[2]

INDICATIONS FOR USE

In gynaecology, the laparoscope is used to allow small operations to be performed in the pelvis or to help make a diagnosis (Table 12.1).

Table 12.1   The indications for gynaecological laparoscopy (from the Royal College of Obstetricians and Gynaecologists Confidential Enquiry into 50 247 operations in 1978)[3]

	Percentage of all laparoscopies
Therapeutic indications	
Sterilization	59.2
Removal of an intrauterine device	1.3
Other indications	0.3
Total	60.8
Diagnostic indications	
Investigation of lower abdominal pain	20.3
Investigation of female infertility	18.0
Other indications	0.8
Total	39.1

OPERATIVE LAPAROSCOPY

The gynaecological operations which can be performed under laparoscopic vision are limited to those which can be done using remote instrumentation. However, the accomplishments of gynaecological laparoscopists are amazing and occasional reports appear of bizarre operations allegedly using a laparoscope and two or more portals of entry into the abdominal cavity. Even appendectomy has been performed under laparoscopic control. For most gynaecologists however, the procedures are limited to sterilization, the division of adhesions, cautery of endometrial lesions and the removal of misplaced intrauterine devices. In those centres where extracorporeal fertilization (in vitro fertilization) is performed, oocyte retrieval is carried out under visual control through the laparoscope. After appropriate ovarian stimulation, four, five or six mature oocytes can be recovered at one operation. With the wider use of high-resolution ultrasound, however, the laparoscopist is giving way to the ultrasonographer in this field.

Sterilization

Sterilization is the commonest single indication for therapeutic laparoscopy in the United Kingdom, about 30 000 operations being performed each year.[3] After proper visualization, each tube is blocked. Electrocautery was the commonest method, using unipolar grounded systems. The high temperature at the end of the active electrode destroys the tube by tissue coagulation and cell death. If a sufficient length of Fallopian tube is destroyed and if there is an area of fibrosis around the burnt area of each tube, it is unlikely to re-canalize spontaneously. However, this unipolar system leaves too little viable tube for future reconstruction to be possible, and it may lead to complications of burns of other tissues such as bladder and bowel. It is now being replaced by bipolar systems. Here a short length of tube is grasped with forceps and the current flows from one jaw of the forceps to the other jaw through the tube.[4] There is less heat generated and consequently a smaller risk of accidental damage to other tissues.

Laparoscopic fulguration is very popular and was recently shown to be the commonest method of sterilization in the United Kingdom. In one year 29 661 sterilisation operations by laparoscopy were performed.[3] Of those where the type of equipment was specified, 23 291 used unipolar fulguration and only 468 used a safer coagulation method. The technique is important. Through the laparoscope, the Fallopian tube is identified and picked up with a grasping forceps. Either a cutting or coagulating current is then applied. Intensive tissue dehydration and charring occurs for about a centimetre on either side of the instrument. Commonly, the operator coagulates each Fallopian tube in two places about 4 cm apart, so there are two areas, each 2 cm long, of destroyed tube. Usually the small segment between the two atrophies and a large gap is left in each tube. Some gynaecologists also divide the charred area through the laparoscope with a remote action scissors but this is becoming less frequent in the 1980s. Wheeless and Thompson report 11 pregnancies in 1000 women with coagulation only (a 1.1% failure rate),[5] whilst Edgerton report 12 pregnancies in 2018 women following coagulation and division (a 0.6% failure rate).[6]

In an effort to achieve greater safety, the low temperature coagulation technique has been applied. In 1974 Semm reported 270 sterilizations by this method without any subsequent pregnancies.[7] With such a small segment of tube destroyed by low-temperature coagulation, it is probably wise to divide the tube in addition.

In the USA and the UK gynaecologists are abandoning electrical destruction of the tubes to achieve sterilization, principally because of the damage that may be caused accidentally to other organs and the litigation which could result. Additionally, increasing consideration is being given to the likelihood of subsequent reversal procedures. This Janus-like philosophy is not held by all gynaecologists and many would advocate that if a couple elect for sterilization it should be considered as a final decision. However, in the Western world many more women are requesting sterilization at a younger age and with smaller families than they did 20 years ago. Mechanical occlusion damages the tube over a shorter area, destroying far less tissue and thus enhancing the possibility of later reanastomosis. Consequently the use of plastic and metal clips applied through the laparoscope to block each tube is becoming more common. A report from the USA on laparoscopic sterilization practice showed that in 1982 21% of procedures used a ring, 4% a clip and 75% were cautery (11% by the unipolar method).

Various types of clip exist, of which the two most commonly used in the UK and the USA are the *Hulka clip,* which has two plastic, toothed jaws hinged by a metal pin and locked closely round the tube by a stainless steel spring (Figure 12.4), and the *Filshie clip,* a plastic clip with a hinge and toothed jaws (Figure 12.5). It has a clasping tooth at the open end which locks the clip closed and so prevents accidental release.

Failure rates of clip sterilization through the laparoscope depend upon the experience of the operator. The most common cause of failure is that the clip does not occlude the tube properly. This may be because it is not fully clicked home or because the Fallopian tube is wider in diameter at the site the clip was applied than the gynaecologist appreciated. Application should be over the narrow isthmial segment, where the tube is less than a centimetre in diameter (Figure 12.5). Clips should not be used when performing a sterilization immediately after a termination of pregnancy for at this

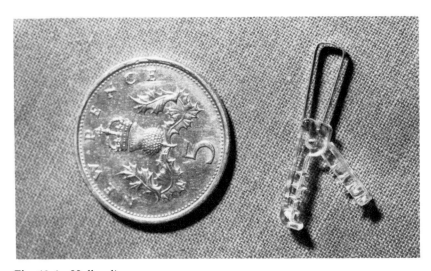

Fig. 12.4 Hulka clip.

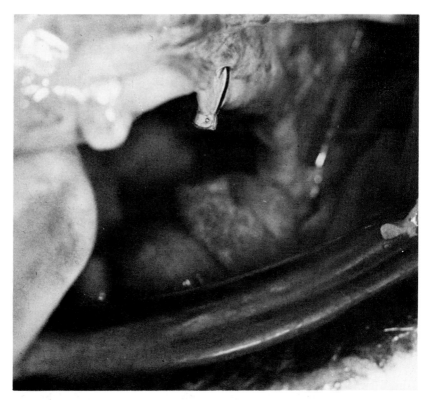

Fig. 12.5   A Filshie clip in place on the Fallopian tube (with thanks to Dr Marcus Filshie).

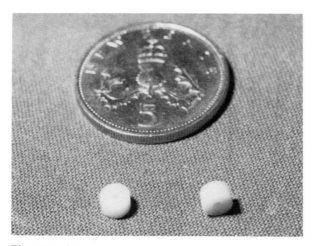

Fig. 12.6   Yoon rings.

time the tube is hypertrophied and the lumen may not be fully occluded by the clip.

Another reason for failure of clip sterilization is that the clip opens slightly some time after application. This might allow passage of sperm but not that of the fertilized ovum; an ectopic pregnancy follows in the lateral part of the Fallopian tube.

Rarely, the clip may cut through the tube so allowing the open lumen of the tube on either side of the clip to rejoin as a fistula.

Hulka et al. reported 24 pregnancies among 907 women sterilized with his clips (a 2.6% failure rate).[9] They considered that if a properly constructed clip were correctly applied to the Fallopian tube, the failure rate would be nearer 0.2%. Filshie et al. reported a failure rate of 0.5% in 540 women sterilized with his titanium silicone rubber clip.[10]

In the last decade, more gynaecologists have used silicon elastic rings. The most common of these is the Fallope or Yoon band (Figure 12.6). The ring is applied with a special tool through the laparoscope and slipped over a knuckle of Fallopian tube producing permanent blockage in two places (Figure 12.7). This method has a low failure rate; for example, Yoon and King reported only three pregnancies in over 900 women sterilized at Johns Hopkins University (a 0.3% failure rate).[11] This method is probably the most popular among younger gynaecologists in the Western world and will be used more frequently in the coming years.

Both mechanical and cautery methods may be applied by the gynaecologist to the wrong area so that structures like the round ligament are inappropriately picked up. For all the above reasons, any woman undergoing sterilization should be warned in advance that there is a small chance of failure (about 1:500 to 1:2000). In the UK a medical indemnity society would find it difficult to defend a gynaecologist if pregnancy followed an operation when the woman had not been told of the risk.

Endometriosis

Endometriosis is the implantation of patches of endometrium outside the uterine cavity. Isolated spots are often seen at laparoscopy, especially in the pouch of Douglas, the back of the uterus and the ovaries. If the gynaecologist thinks these are associated with symptoms, they can be coagulated with a small button or blade cautery. Whilst such actions are relatively safe on the back of the uterus and over the ovarian surfaces, care is needed with deposits on the rectum or on the side walls of the pelvis since perforation of the

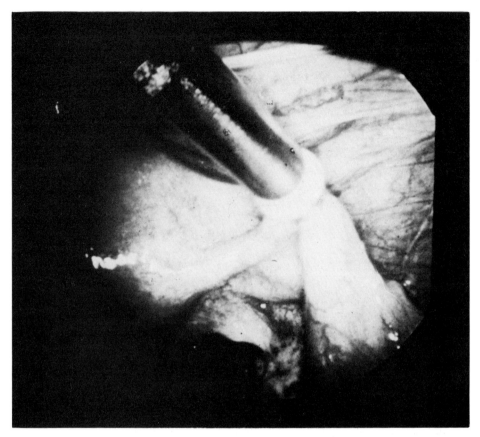

Fig. 12.7   A laparoscopic view of a Yoon ring in place on the Fallopian tube.

rectum and damage to other structures like the ureter may follow too enthusiastic cautery.

Adhesiolysis

Small adhesions considered to be the cause of problems can be divided at laparoscopy with hooked scissors but the gynaecologist must be able to cauterize immediately via the laparoscope if bleeding follows.

Intrauterine devices

Intrauterine devices may perforate the uterus or upper cervix during insertion. If this is suspected they can be detected at laparoscopy and removed by this route, provided they have not been in the peritoneal cavity so long that they are bound to the underlying tissues by adhesions. In such circumstances laparoscopic removal could cause tears. The copper-bearing devices (Copper 7 or T) have a greater tendency to stimulate adhesions than the plain plastic devices. If omentum covers the location fluoroscopic equipment can guide the operator.[12]

DIAGNOSTIC LAPAROSCOPY

In the last ten years laparoscopy has made a great difference to the diagnosis of both acute and chronic pelvic pain. A possible leaking ectopic pregnancy at the ampullary end of the Fallopian tube can be rapidly confirmed or ruled out, so saving days of patient's time in the hospital. The causes of chronic pain are now being diagnosed more precisely; endometriosis is found more frequently and small adhesions can be treated. Even if nothing is seen, laparoscopy is advantageous to the woman. She can then be reassured that there is no condition present which needs surgical treatment – a very helpful statement to many patients, who will often then tolerate lesser pain until it passes away by sublimation.

The other important use for diagnostic laparoscopy is the investigation of female infertility. Tubal blockage and damage is found in 15% of couples, for whom a cause of infertility can be specified. Whilst the lumen of the tube can be silhouetted with radiopaque dyes at hysterosalpingography, laparoscopy not only allows tubal patency to be assessed but also enables other features in the pelvis to be examined, such as kinking of the tube, fimbrial damage or ovarian adhesions. The presence of a corpus luteum is good evidence of current ovulation. When dye is injected along the Fallopian tube, the volume insufflated before the dye appears at the fimbriated end should be noted. A better prognosis is associated with appearance at low volumes (under 10 ml).

If tubal surgery is contemplated to reverse a previous sterilization operation, *it is mandatory that the gynaecologist who will do the repair performs a preliminary laparoscopy himself or herself in order to assess the prospects for successful anastomosis.* Sometimes so much tube has been destroyed at the first operation that it would be foolish to proceed: other methods of resolving the problem such as adoption or extracorporeal fertilization should be reassessed.

Another laparoscopic technique that may be used in the diagnosis of infertility and amenorrhoea is ovarian biopsy. The wider use of functional tests of ovarian stimulation by gonadotrophins and gonadotrophin-releasing hormones has greatly reduced the need for biopsy but it can still be of help if the presence of primordial follicles is in doubt in primary amenorrhoea or premature ovarian failure (Figure 12.8). If biopsy is attempted, a reasonable sample of tissue must be sent to the pathologist. At least $5\,mm^3$ is needed: a scraping from the surface is not good enough. Ovarian biopsy at laparoscopy can be difficult, for the woman who needs this diagnostic test often has smooth mobile ovaries. These slide away from conventional biopsy forceps, offering little grip for the forceps' jaws on their surface. The screw-home punch devised by Palmer (or Frangenheim beak punch forceps) is recommended, rather than the miniature crocodile forceps often provided by many manufacturers in their laparoscopy kits.

The follow-up of women treated for ovarian cancer may involve laparoscopy. With the wider use of powerful combinations of cytotoxic drugs, more women are surviving and the philosophy of second-look (and even third-, fourth- and fifth-look) examination is spreading. Some gynaecological oncologists consider that laparoscopy provides too limited an examination – they complain that parts

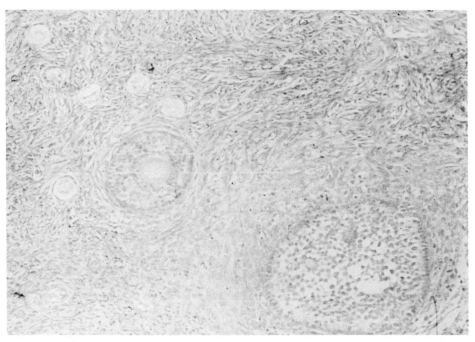

(a)

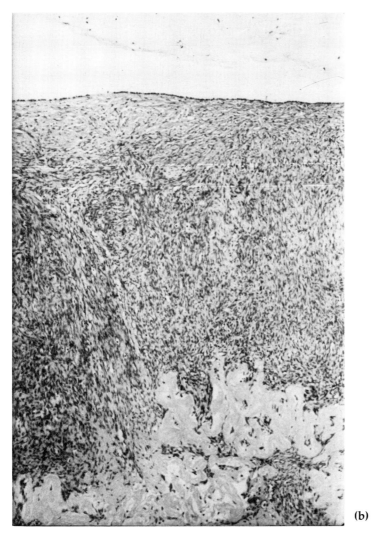

(b)

Fig. 12.8 (a) Normal ovarian tissue showing numerous primary and secondary follicles. (b) Primary ovarian failure with a dearth of follicles (with acknowledgements to Dr Margaret Burke).

of the pelvis, the paracolic gutters and the diaphragmatic surface of the liver are not well seen, and so they employ repeated laparotomies. This may reflect inexperience with the laparoscope, because with patience and appropriate adjustments to the angle of the operating table, these areas can usually be seen. Adhesions after earlier radical surgery may present problems but they should not be obstacles to successful laparoscopy for the experienced operator. The woman who has had radical surgery for carcinoma of the ovary, greatly appreciates having a re-look laparoscopy rather than a repeat laparotomy.

THE PROCEDURE

The performance of gynaecological laparoscopy is best learnt in the operating theatre with an experienced operator, and this chapter will be confined to principles. Gynaecological laparoscopy is not a minor procedure. It may use narrow-bore instruments and work through small incisions, but it is not an operation to be delegated to the less skilled junior colleague at the end of the operating list. The hazards in the hands of the unskilled are great: it is much safer to leave, if necessary, an unsupervised junior to perform a laparotomy than a laparoscopy. The wider exposure will allow the less experienced to deal with any problems they may create.

As with other operations, preoperative preparation of the patient is important. Specifically, the anaesthetist must be involved. Gynaecological laparoscopy can be performed under local anaesthesia, backed up by pethidine (meperidine) and diazepam but in the Western world this is rarely used. The unpleasant sensation produced by stretch of peritoneum cannot be adequately covered by local anaesthesia. Epidural anaesthesia is of little value since the site of application necessary to affect the entire peritoneum would be so high that it would interfere with intercostal nerves and affect respiration. Most commonly, a general anaesthetic is employed and, since this has its own pitfalls, skilled help is required for effective relaxation and intubation in 90% of patients.[3] As the operation requires an experienced gynaecologist, so the anaesthetic must be administered by a skilled anaesthetist.[13]

In the operating theatre the anaesthetized patient is placed in the oblique lithotomy position to allow the gynaecologist and an assistant to work simultaneously from the vaginal and abdominal approaches. The thighs must not be flexed onto the abdominal wall as they would be in the full lithotomy position used for a dilatation and curettage. The bladder is emptied by an indwelling catheter.

The optimum incision is in the subumbilical region, with a slightly curved 1–2 cm cut following the lower fold of the umbilicus. This is deepened to open the rectus sheath. Other approaches may be lower in the midline, avoiding the bladder, or in one or other iliac fossa avoiding the inferior epigastric vessels (Figure 12.9). The anterior

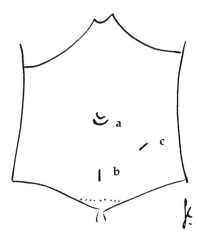

Fig. 12.9 Sites of incision for gynaecological laparoscopy:
(a) subumbilical;
(b) suprapubic;
(c) lateral to rectus muscle.

abdominal wall is usually picked up in a big pinch so that the Veress needle can be introduced and the abdominal cavity distended with gas.

During insufflation intra-abdominal pressure is monitored, keeping it below 20–25 mmHg (2.7–3.3 kPa). Whilst air could be used, nitrogen, which makes up 80% of air, dissolves slowly so that the woman has more discomfort for 24–48 hours afterwards. Carbon dioxide is more soluble and is the commonest insufflating gas; absorption across the peritoneum can occur during the operation but acidaemia, with its accompanying increased risk of cardiac arrhythmia is rare. If the woman has a normal respiratory system and her respiration is being managed by a competent anaesthetist, she can deal easily with the slightly increased load of hydrogen ions.

Fears of acid–base imbalance due to carbon dioxide absorption led for a time to insufflation with another commonly available gas, nitrous oxide. However, if after a minor prick with a needle any of the organic gases from the alimentary tract should escape into the peritoneal cavity, *a powerful explosive mixture can result; several cases of fatal intra-abdominal explosions have been reported when cautery sparking occurred in this gas mixture.*[14] It must be remembered, however, that should local anaesthetic have to be used for laparoscopy, nitrous oxide is less irritating to the peritoneum than carbon dioxide and is safe if no electrical cautery is involved in the operation.

When a dome of gas has been generated between the abdominal wall and its contents, the woman is tipped head down to about 25° from the horizontal (reversed Trendelenberg); a steeper angle is not needed. Usually 2–3 l of the insufflating gas are required in the first phase and the trocar with its sheath is then introduced through the same subumbilical wound. For added safety, the operator aims the trocar at the sacral promontory, thus trying to avoid both the intestinal contents, which should have moved towards the posterior part of the upper abdomen, and the bifurcation of the aorta, which, with the confluence of the common iliac veins, is about 4 cm above the promontory.

The pre-warmed laparoscope is introduced through the trocar sleeve, and a low flow of insufflating gas continued through a side channel to allow for the loss of gas by leakage and absorption. Viewing the lateral pelvic organs is helped by the manipulation of mobile structures with a solid probe introduced either through a separate incision or down the channel of an operating laparoscope. The ovary needs inspection on all surfaces, not just that which faces the laparoscope. The posterior pelvis and pouch of Douglas are best seen when the uterus is elevated by the assistant working at the vaginal end.

Sometimes, when the telescope is inserted, the Veress needle is seen to have passed extraperitoneally, never having left the space behind the rectus muscles. Gas has expanded this loose area and the view obtained is of strands of connective tissue and glistening fat globules. The operator must start again, introducing the needle at a steeper angle or, if the patient is obese, using a longer needle.

After assessing the genital organs, the gynaecologist may wish to view areas outside the pelvis. This is easily done by tilting the table head up or laterally to examine the paracolic or sub-diaphragmatic spaces.

After the laparoscopy is finished, the telescope is removed and the gas is allowed to escape through the opened cannula. There is no need to pummel the abdominal wall: gentle pressure with the flat of the hand will ensure expulsion of the maximum volume – about a half of that insufflated. Although carbon dioxide is theoretically more soluble than nitrous oxide, I reported no significant difference in the proportion of the two gases returned in a large, randomized study.[15] The wound is closed with a single Michel clip, and a small non-occlusive dry dressing completes the operation.

THE RISKS OF GYNAECOLOGICAL LAPAROSCOPY

The known risks of any operation do not rest only upon the skills of the operator, but also on the ability of the reporting methods to gather accurate information. Most studies reporting hazards are of a limited size, relating to one or two hospitals and to a few

Table 12.2   The complications of gynaecological laparoscopy (from the
RCOG Confidential Enquiry into 50 247 operations in 1978)[3]

	No. of cases	Rate per 1000 laparoscopies
Anaesthetic complications		
Anaesthetist	38	0.8
Cardiac arrest	9	0.2
Cardiac arrhythmias	20	0.4
Failed procedures		
Failed laparoscopy	375	7.5
Failed abdominal insufflation	178	3.5
Failed vaginal insufflation	2	0.0
Burns		
Bowel burn	27	0.5
Skin burn	13	0.3
Other burns	10	0.2
Direct trauma		
Bowel	90	1.8
Urinary tract	11	0.2
Damage to pelvic organs	172	3.4
Haemorrhage		
Abdominal wall	125	2.5
Pelvic blood vessels and tubal mesentery	134	2.7
Pelvic sidewall and ovarian vessels	43	0.9
Mesentery of bowel	54	1.1
Infection		
Abdominal wound	26	0.5
Pelvic infection	25	0.5
Chest infection	11	0.2
Urinary tract	24	0.5
Other complications		
Chest pain	13	0.3
Lost foreign body	29	0.6
Damage to pelvic organs not due to laparoscopy procedures	132	2.6
Pulmonary embolism	8	0.2
Deep vein thrombosis	10	0.2
Other	156	3.1
Late complications	41	0.8
Deaths	4	0.1

gynaecologists of some experience. Often the very fact that they have bothered to write up a series shows a particular interest, so they probably have some special skills in the subject and hence a lower complication rate. Further, their reports of complicated cases partly reflect their larger experience.

The range of reported complications after gynaecological laparoscopy seems wide. Johnson reported an overall complication rate of 43 per 1000,[16] whilst Paterson and Grimwald reported a major complication rate of 13 per 1000 in a review of 600 laparoscopic sterilizations.[17] In 1976–77 the Royal College of Obstetricians and Gynaecologists (RCOG) carried out a confidential enquiry into over 50000 gynaecological laparoscopies during that period, reporting a gross rate of all complications of 34 per 1000.[3] The natures of the complications are listed in Table 12.2.

The rates were found to be highest in sterilization laparoscopy procedures – 40 per 1000 compared with 30 per 1000 in the diagnostic category.

Seniority of the operator

In the RCOG study, the seniority of the gynaecologist performing the operation was recorded, together with whether or not there was supervision. The group with the highest complication rate of all was the clinical assistants but the total number of doctors in this group was small. For laparoscopic sterilizations, the lowest complication rate was amongst the consultant surgeons – 34 per 1000 compared with 48 per 1000 for senior registrars, 42 for registrars and 54 for senior house surgeons. The complication rates were generally higher in the supervised procedures – 50 per 1000 for supervised cases compared with an overall incidence of 44 per 1000 for non-supervised cases.

It is difficult to draw the conclusion that there was a direct cause-and-effect relationship: it may be that the more senior people performed the more difficult operations and therefore might have expected a higher complication rate. Furthermore, those operations performed by supervised juniors may also have been those in which trouble was anticipated, necessitating the presence of a senior gynaecologist.

The nature of the complications

Complications were reported in 1818 women out of the 50247 who had a gynaecological operation – an overall rate of 36.2 per 1000. In 91 patients there were two or more complications. Anaesthetic complications occurred in 38; perhaps unfairly, cardiac arrest and arrhythmia were grouped into this category. There were respectively 9 and 20 of these.

Laparoscopy failed on the first attempt in 7.5 per 1000. This failure rate may seem high, but it should be borne in mind that this was a confidential enquiry in which surgeons were not at risk of any retribution as a consequence of their reports. In most cases, the surgeon repeated the procedure and succeeded on a second occasion under the same anaesthetic.

More seriously, direct trauma to the bowel was reported in 90 women, most of whom underwent laparotomy to inspect and sometimes repair the bowel. Damage to other pelvic organs occurred in 172. This was mostly to the uterus, a problem of little significance. The bladder was damaged in 11, in 9 of whom it was insufflated with gas. Burns of the bowel occurred in 27 women; all cases were serious, necessitating intestinal resection.

A much higher number of cases were reported with haemorrhage, the most serious being those to the pelvic side wall and mesentery of the bowel (43 and 54 cases respectively). Haemorrhage from the tubal mesentery (134 cases) can usually be readily dealt with by cautery or clip on the bleeding vessel, either method being possible using a laparoscope.

The incidence of infection is probably under-reported in the RCOG study for data were only collected as long as the woman was in hospital (one or two days usually). These figures are lower than the ones often quoted in the American literature, where the attending gynaecologist is usually involved in the care of the woman even after she has left the hospital.

The nature of the complications was examined in relation to the status of the gynaecologist and this breakdown followed the same pattern as has been previously described. Consultants generally had the lowest rate of complications, except for trauma to the bowel, where all seniorities seemed to be at risk; this may reflect the fact that some of the trauma occurs with the first insufflation with the Veress needle, which is performed blind.

The different sterilization techniques were compared. Complications were not very frequent, but among the commonly used methods the application of rings or bands was associated with a markedly higher complication rate than that of cautery. An even higher rate of complication was demonstrated if the tube was both cut and coagulated.

Longer term failure rates of sterilization (that is, pregnancy occurring after sterilization) were not examined in this study, which was purely short-term. Failure rates referred to previously in this chapter have been derived from other sources.

It is usually considered that laparoscopy performed in relation to pregnancy produces a higher rate of complications, and so it is conventional teaching not to do sterilization operations at the same time as termination of pregnancy. No such increase in complication rates was found in the RCOG study. However, one of the problems of such an operation is that the occlusion of the tube may not be complete. The hormonal changes of pregnancy make the Fallopian tube bulkier and more vascular. In consequence, a clip may not properly occlude the lumen and a ring could spring off postoperatively.

The type of laparoscope used made little difference to the complication rates in the diagnostic group, but among women who were sterilized the single portal route was associated with a complication rate of 60 per 1000 whereas the multiple portal route produced a rate of only 37 per 1000. The numbers of women involved made these data significantly different ($P < 0.05$). It may be that the more limited vision provided to the gynaecologist was associated with complications.

Four deaths were reported in the enquiry, a mortality rate of 0.08 per 1000 cases. It must be stressed that with events as rare as this a single case makes an apparently large alteration in the rate. One death was associated with an infertility investigation and the other three with sterilizing operations. Three had been performed by consultants and the fourth by a senior house officer under the supervision of the consultant. Similarly, the anaesthetic was given by a consultant in three cases and a medical assistant under supervision in the fourth. One death followed a proven gas embolism, two resulted from cardiac arrest that could not be reversed and the fourth followed perforation of small bowel leading to infection.

This chapter has merely outlined the complications of gynaecological laparoscopy. For details readers are referred to the original RCOG report.[3]

A review of complications in 1982 was performed by the American Association of Gynecological Laparoscopists: 125 560 sterilization operations were reviewed.[8] The report showed a rate of major complications requiring hospitalization of 1.45 per thousand cases. Bowel injury accounted for 0.42 per 1000, haemorrhage 0.45 per 1000 and pelvic infection 0.45 per 1000. These figures are much lower than those reported in the RCOG enquiry but allowance must be made for the fact that the American enquiry was a voluntary one performed by the members of a specialist gynaecological laparoscopy society who had extra interest and could be expected to have extra experience and skills in the subject while the RCOG enquiry was of all seniorities of doctors, including those under training as well as trained gynaecologists.

CONCLUSIONS

All operations have risks and thoughtful surgeons weigh these against the advantages; they then recommend to individual patients those procedures in which the merits outweigh the hazards. Gynaecological laparoscopy is very useful in the diagnosis of pelvic pathology and for performing certain limited pelvic procedures. If used with care, by trained gynaecologists, it is of immense help to women with pelvic and reproductive conditions.

ACKNOWLEDGEMENTS

My thanks are due to the Royal College of Obstetricians and Gynaecologists who have allowed me to quote extensively from their Confidential Enquiry.[3] I am also grateful to Dr Margaret Burke of the Pathology Department of St George's Hospital Medical School who provided me with the two photographs of ovarian tissue biopsies.

REFERENCES

1   Short, A.R. (1925) *Br. med. J. ii:* 254–256.
2   The Royal College of Obstetricians and Gynaecologists Working Party on Gynaecological Laparoscopy (1982) *A Review of Laparoscopy Equipment Available in the United Kingdom.* London: Royal College of Obstetricians and Gynaecologists.
3   Chamberlain, G. & Brown, J.C. (1978) *Gynaecological Laparoscopy. The Report of a Working Party in a Confidential Enquiry of Gynaecological Laparoscopy.* London: Royal College of Obstetricians and Gynaecologists.
4   Rioux, J. (1974) True bipolar electro-surgery for tubal sterilization by laparoscopy. In *Gynecological Laparoscopy*, Phillips, J. & Keith, L. (eds). New York: Stratton Intercontinental.
5   Wheeless, C.R. & Thompson, B.H. (1973) Laparoscopy sterilization – a review of 3600 cases. *Obstet. Gynec.* 42: 751–758.
6   Edgerton, W.D. (1974) Laparoscopy in the community hospital. In *Gynaecological Laparoscopy*, Phillips, J. & Keith, L. (eds). New York: Stratton Intercontinental.
7   Semm, K. (1974) Tubal sterilization. In *Gynaecological Laparoscopy*, Phillips, J. & Keith, L. (eds). New York: Stratton Intercontinental.

8   Phillips, J.M., Hulka, J.F. & Peterson, H. (1984) American Association of Gynecologic Laparoscopists 1982 Membership Survey. *J. repro. Med. 29:* 592–594.

9   Hulka, J.F., Omran, K., Phillips, J.M. et al. (1975) Sterilization by spring clip. *Fert. & Steril. 26:* 1122–1131.

10 Filshie, G.M., Casey, D., Pogmore, J. et al. (1981) The Tetaneum silicone rubber clip for female sterilization. *Br. J. Obstet. & Gynaec. 88:* 655–662.

11 Yoon, I.B. & King, T.M. (1976) The laparoscopic fallope ring procedure. In *Advances in Female Sterilization Technology*, Sciama, J. et al. (eds). Hagerstown, Maryland: Harper & Row.

12 Brooks, P.G., Berci, G., Lawrence, A., Slypian, P. & Wade, M. (1972) Removal of intra-abdominal intra-uterine contraceptive devices through a peritoneoscope with the use of intra-operative fluoroscopy to aid localisation. *Am. J. Obstet. Gynec. 113:*

13 Calverley, R.K. & Jenkins, L.C. (1973) The anaesthetic management of pelvic laparoscopy. *Can. Anaesth. Soc. J. 20:* 279–286.

14 El Kady, A. & Abdl el Razek, K. (1976) Intraperitoneal explosion during female sterilization by laparoscopy electro-coagulation. *Int. J. Gynaec. & Obstet. 14:* 487–488.

15 Chamberlain, G. (1984) The fate of insufflated gases. *Br. J. Obstet. Gynaec. 91:* 367–370.

16 Johnson, C.E. (1976) Laparoscopy (700 cases). *Clin. Obstet. Gynec. 19:* 707–719.

17 Paterson, P.J. & Grimwade, J.C. (1973) A review of 600 laparoscopic sterilizations. *Aust. N.Z. J Obstet. Gynaec. 13:* 165–168.

13
Complications of Laparoscopy

Laparoscopy is a safe and well tolerated procedure in the hands of an experienced and skilled operator. The reported mortality of several large series of non-gynaecological laparoscopy is small: it varies from 0 to 0.3% (Table 13.1). To some extent the morbidity and mortality are dependent on the age, general condition and coexisting cardiorespiratory disease etc, and comparisons between different series are difficult. The common complications are usually of a minor nature but a few are life-threatening. The overriding factors in the causation of

Table 13.1 Reported mortality for non-gynaecological laparoscopy

Published series	Year	Number of patients	Number of deaths	Mortality (%)
Ruddock	1957	2500	3	0.1
Zoeckler	1958	1000	3	0.3
Bruhl	1966	63845	19	0.03
Villardel et al.	1968	1455	2	0.1
Wildhirt et al.	1969	10500	2	0.02
Look	1972	2900	1	0.03
Tadaki et al.	1974	24133	4	0.01
Cuschieri	1980	1416	0	—
Berci and Jensen	1982	800	0	—
Zimmerman	1982	1000	0	—

the serious iatrogenic injuries is faulty technique arising from inexperience or lack of proper training. It is surprising that laparoscopy features little in surgical and gastroenterological clinical training programmes. In this respect gynaecologists are way ahead of surgeons and gastroenterologists but then laparoscopy is an essential and commonly used procedure in modern gynaecology. This chapter reviews the morbidity of the procedure, with an emphasis on the prevention of complications and the appropriate course of action in the event of their occurrence.

RISK FACTORS

Aside from faulty technique and inexperience, the risk of complications is enhanced in the presence of certain well recognized circumstances and an awareness of these is essential to the conduct of safe laparoscopy.

Systemic factors

These relate to coexisting cardio-respiratory disorders and deficiencies of the clotting mechanism. Laparoscopy is best avoided for three months after a myocardial infarction. In patients with ischaemic heart disease, the procedure should be performed under general anaesthesia with endotracheal intubation and continuous monitoring by a skilled anaesthetist. Abnormalities of the clotting mechanism, revealed as a prolongation of the prothrombin time must be corrected before the procedure by intramuscular vitamin K therapy and by the administration of fresh frozen plasma if the prothrombin time remains elevated despite vitamin K therapy. Laparoscopy can be performed in the presence of moderate to severe thrombocytopenia. In this situation it is best to hold platelet transfusion in reserve unless it becomes necessary because of bleeding. If a liver biopsy is considered necessary, the biopsy site must be observed to have stopped bleeding after compression by the palpating probe. Should bleeding continue haemostasis is then achieved by diathermy coagulation.

Previous surgery

The risk of organ damage is enhanced in the presence of adhesions from previous surgical interventions and these cases should not be attempted by the beginner. The techniques to be followed in these cases are outlined in Chapter 5.

Ascites

It is not sufficiently appreciated that in the presence of ascites the gas-filled intestinal loops tend to float on the surface of the fluid and are more liable to injury by the Veress needle or laparoscopic trocar. In addition, the abdominal wall in these patients is weak as a result of muscular atrophy and therefore there is a tendency for the needle or trocar suddenly to jerk into the peritoneal cavity.

Obesity

Marked obesity enhances the technical difficulty and impairs inspection of the peritoneal contents. Indeed, the procedure should not be undertaken in the morbidly obese. In any event, in most of these patients the trocar does not reach the peritoneal cavity. The risk of gas extravasation into the abdominal wall, mesentery or omentum is increased in obese patients.

Organ distension

This includes a full urinary bladder, which accounts for the majority of penetrating injuries to this organ during laparoscopy. All patients should void or preferably be catheterized before the procedure. The same consideration applies to a distended stomach from pyloric obstruction.

Interventional therapeutic procedures

The risks of both bleeding and organ damage are enhanced with biopsy, cholangiography and various gynaecological therapeutic procedures. Adequate training in these specific procedures is essential. The postoperative monitoring and care must of necessity be more rigorous and prolonged than in patients who have only a diagnostic inspection. All patients who have a needle biopsy of the liver must be kept in bed for at least 12 hours. This period is longer (1–2 days) for patients who have a splenic biopsy. Once again it must be stressed that a splenic biopsy is a hazardous procedure and should not be attempted lightly.

PATHOPHYSIOLOGY OF THE ARTIFICIAL PNEUMOPERITONEUM

The creation of a pneumoperitoneum is accompanied by cardiovascular, pH and blood gas changes which are dependent on the nature and amount of gas insufflated, the level of intra-abdominal pressure reached, the type of anaesthesia employed and the adequacy of ventilation. An understanding of the pathophysiological changes consequent on the artificially induced pneumoperitoneum is therefore essential to the conduct of safe laparoscopy. With appropriate technique, adequate instrumentation, careful, pressure-controlled insufflation and patient monitoring, these changes are minimized and serious life-threatening complications can be largely averted.

Early studies[10] indicated that an elevation of intra-abdominal pressure to 10–15mmHg (1.3–2.0kPa) following air insufflation caused a rise in both the venous and arterial pressure. The extent of upward displacement of the diaphragm for a given level of intraabdominal pressure varies with each subject.[11] When appreciable, the resulting cardiac displacement is accompanied by definite ECG changes. These include changes in the QRS complex with deviation of the electrical axis to the left, an increase in the amplitude of R_1 and a decreased amplitude of R_3. Inversion of T_3 is observed when the pneumoperitoneum is complete.

The changes accompanying insufflation of the peritoneal cavity with CO_2 are well documented.[11–13] The main advantage of this gas is that it does not support combustion and this accounts for its popularity and widespread use. CO_2 insufflation results in a rise in the central venous and systemic arterial pressures. The rise in the blood pressure is mainly due to a sympathetic drive consequent on the hypercarbia and to a lesser extent on the increased pressure on the abdominal aorta. When the intra-abdominal pressure exceeds 20 mmHg (2.7 kPa), the CVP and blood pressure fall, in association with a diminished cardiac output. There is a good correlation between the volume of CO_2 insufflated and the fall in the cardiac output.[14] The average fall in cardiac output during CO_2 pneumoperitoneum is 0.5–0.6 l/min – a 16–17% drop.[15] Muscle relaxation during general endotracheal anaesthesia, as well as facilitating the examination, keeps the rise in the intra-abdominal pressure within acceptable limits and ensures adequate ventilation.

Arrhythmias are common with CO_2 insufflation. The most frequent is bradycardia, which results from reflex vagal stimulation due to stretching of the peritoneal surface or local irritation by CO_2. Premedication with atropine prevents the bradycardia.[16] Other more serious arrhythmias include bigeminal rhythm, ventricular ectopic beats and ventricular tachycardia. These are mainly due to inadequate ventilation especially when the patient is in the Trendelenburg position.[16]

CO_2 insufflation is also accompanied by a rise in the arterial PCO_2 and a fall in the arterial pH and PO_2.[4,17] In addition, the serum chloride level drops owing to a shift of the chloride ions into the RBCs in exchange for bicarbonate ions consequent on the hypercarbia. The respiratory acidosis manifested by a raised PCO_2, fall in pH and an unchanged bicarbonate and base excess is usually mild or absent if the procedure is carried out under general anaesthesia with controlled ventilation and is more pronounced if the patient is allowed to breathe spontaneously.[18] The rise in the PCO_2 is due to absorption of CO_2 from the peritoneal cavity but may also result from impaired ventilation due to narcotic sedation when the procedure is carried out under local anaesthesia.

Although N_2O is not inflammable, it supports combustion. This is the only disadvantage of using this gas in laparoscopy since diathermy coagulation cannot be used during the procedure. In all other respects it is a better alternative to CO_2 and is not accompanied by a significant blood pH and blood gas changes. The cardiovascular changes, especially the blood pressure, return rapidly to normal after desufflation as there is no significant sympathetic drive during N_2O insufflation.[17] There is a documented lower incidence of cardiac arrhythmias with N_2O insufflation.[19] Although N_2O is not absorbed as rapidly as CO_2 from the peritoneal surface, its absorption is sufficiently rapid to avoid prolonged postoperative distention and discomfort. In a blind study on discomfort during laparoscopy under local anaesthesia, N_2O was observed to be more comfortable than CO_2 as perceived by both the patient and the physician and by objective assessment of the degree of abdominal splinting.[20]

Practical implications

All patients undergoing laparoscopy should have continuous monitoring of the blood pressure and ECG irrespective of the type of anaesthesia used. In patients with a tendency to cardiac failure, the central venous pressure should also be monitored. High-risk patients with cardio-respiratory disease should have the procedure under general endotracheal anaesthesia using muscle relaxants and controlled ventilation with a gas mixture containing at least 50% oxygen.

The amount of gas insufflated should be kept at a minimum. Insufflation should be slow and *the intra-abdominal pressure should not exceed 20 mmHg (2.7 kPa)*. Premedication with atropine is advisable when CO_2 is used as the insufflating agent. The onset of any cardiac arrhythmias is an indication to stop insufflation. If the changes are rapidly reversed, the procedure may continue with careful monitoring.

CARDIAC COMPLICATIONS

Serious cardiac complications apart from arrhythmias are rare: *cardiac failure* and *cardiac arrest* due to ventricular fibrillation occur at a rate of 0.2 per 1000 laparoscopies.[21] The risk factors include pre-existing ischaemic heart disease and inadequate ventilation due to diaphragmatic splinting, particularly in the Trendelenburg position with the patient breathing spontaneously. Cardiac failure occurs early in the procedure when the insufflation causes a rise in the central venous pressure in patients with incipient heart failure before the procedure. This stresses the need for CVP monitoring in these patients.

Gas embolism

This rare but potentially fatal complication is the main reason for avoiding air as the insufflation agent. In animal experiments volumes of 0.25 ml/kg of air injected intravenously are lethal whereas much larger volumes of CO_2, equivalent to 1 litre in a human, can be injected before the cardiac output falls significantly.[22] Nitrous oxide is slightly less soluble than CO_2 in the blood. Gas embolism with CO_2 or N_2O is very rare. Accurate data on its incidence are difficult to ascertain since the criteria for diagnosis vary considerably in the literature and definite diagnosis can only be obtained by the confirmation of gas bubbles at surgery or postmortem. However, the use of a precordial Doppler ultrasound probe for detection of the bubbles has recently been reported.[23] Embolism of large amounts of gas leads to cardiovascular collapse due to right ventricular outflow tract obstruction. In cases of gas embolism reported in the literature, evidence of direct vascular injury and injection of gas is often absent.[24] In some cases penetration of the uterus by the Veress needle suggests direct injection of gas into a uterine vein. Rupture of an intraperitoneal vein with consequent direct entry of CO_2 into the vascular system because of the increased intra-abdominal pressure has been suggested as the mechanism responsible when no vascular or solid organ injury is discernible.[25] One report implicated possible CO_2 absorption from an inflamed appendix.[24]

If gas embolism is suspected, the patient should be immediately placed in the left lateral position with the head down to minimize the right outflow tract obstruction. Scanning with a precordial Doppler probe will reveal a mill-wheel murmur. A Swan Ganz catheter should be inserted for monitoring of the pulmonary artery pressure and the pulmonary capillary wedge pressure.

PULMONARY COMPLICATIONS

The commonest complication is *bronchopulmonary aspiration* of refluxed gastric contents. Absolute starvation for 12 hours does not abolish this risk since the raised intra-abdominal pressure is such as to overcome the anti-reflux mechanism at the cardio-oesophageal junction at least in some patients when reflux of the basal gastric juice occurs. Endotracheal anaesthesia minimizes this risk although bronchopulmonary aspiration can occur either before or shortly after endobronchial intubation. When severe, the chest X-ray shows diffuse shadowing due to pulmonary oedema. Treatment includes bronchial toilet, diuretics, short-term ventilatory support and antibiotics.

Pulmonary embolism is extremely rare and is largely confined to therapeutic gynaecological laparoscopy (see Chapter 12). Thus for general diagnostic laparoscopy specific prophylaxis against deep vein thrombosis is unwarranted although the use of TED stockings and early ambulation should be encouraged.

Pneumothorax and mediastinal emphysema is a rare but well recognized complication of laparoscopy. The mediastinal emphysema is usually self-limiting and of short duration when CO_2 and N_2O are used. Intercostal underwater seal drainage is necessary for the pneumothorax.

PENETRATING INJURIES

These are usually the result of faulty technique and inexperience. Other risk factors include adhesions from previous surgical intervention and distended hollow viscera (full bladder, distended stomach, colon etc.). They are caused by the Veress needle or the laparoscopic trocar. The commonest injuries are vascular: parietal vessels, mesenteric veins, iliac vessels and rarely the aorta or vena cava. The hollow visceral organs which are most at risk are the urinary bladder and loops of small intestine.

Needle injuries are rare if the protocol outlined in Chapter 5 is followed carefully, with special emphasis on trial aspiration and close attention to the intra-abdominal pressure during insufflation. Trocar injuries can be largely avoided by adopting the right technique of trocar insertion with careful selection of site and avoidance of sudden thrusts during penetration of the abdominal wall. The technique outlined in Chapter 5 will obviate the vast majority of serious injuries. It emphasizes the controlled drilling–pressing action with a safety stop once resistance to further advancement of the trocar is encountered.

The management of these injuries depends on their severity. Minor vascular injuries caused by the Veress needle result in a haematoma. In this situation the needle position is changed, laparoscopic inspection is continued and the haematoma is observed for several minutes. Enlargement of the haematoma or development of hypotension are indications for immediate surgical exploration. Otherwise, the patient is observed closely after the procedure.

Major vascular injury is indicated by severe hypotension from hypovolaemic shock. No attempt should be made to inspect the peritoneal cavity and the laparoscopic instruments should be left in situ. Volume replacement with a colloidal solution and blood should be started together with an immediate exploration by a competent general or vascular surgeon.

Injuries to hollow viscera caused by the Veress needle should be recognized early. If they are not, the insufflation results in an asymmetric pneumoperitoneum and a marked rise in the pressure. The needle should be withdrawn and reinserted, after which insufflation is recommended. Careful inspection of the site of injury is essential to ascertain the size of the tear, the amount, if any, of leakage of bowel contents and any associated injury. If the lesion is less than about 2 mm in size and little or no leakage is observed, the patient is treated conservatively with nasogastric suction and antibiotics. These lesions heal spontaneously provided they are not associated with mesenteric vascular damage which may lead to necrosis and perforation.

All trocar injuries to intra-abdominal organs are serious and require immediate surgical exploration.

MINOR COMPLICATIONS

Some of these complications, such as bruising around stab wounds, are common and are often overlooked. Postoperative pain referred to the shoulder is far less common when CO_2 or N_2O is used instead of air. None the less it still occurs and is due to irritation of the diaphragm by minor oozing of blood into the peritoneal cavity. Certain minor complications deserve special mention since they may lead to more serious sequelae if they are overlooked or cause considerable distress to the patients. These include extravasation of gas causing surgical emphysema, wound infection, leakage of ascitic fluid and omental prolapse.

Extravasation of gas

The most common error which occurs during insufflation is the creation of a pre-peritoneal or intra-abdominal omental emphysema.

Less commonly the gas is inadvertently insufflated between the leaves of the mesentery. Although the gas is rapidly absorbed, the emphysema, if not recognized early on, may considerably impair visualization of the peritoneal cavity and its contents. This complication arises from faulty insertion of the Veress needle. The operator should become aware of this eventuality if he observes a high initial pressure on the intra-abdominal pressure gauge or slow infusion of gas which is reflected by a low position of the flow-meter ball. Sometimes the insufflation starts with a low pressure reading, suggesting that the tip of the needle is free within the peritoneal cavity, but the pressure then increases rapidly. This indicates insufflation of gas into a confined space, creating a balloon effect. When recognized, the insufflation is stopped, the needle is withdrawn and an alternative site for its reinsertion is selected. One must then ensure that the needle can be moved through an arc without any rise in the intra-abdominal pressure.

Wound infection

Despite the well demonstrated difficulties in sterilizing the umbilicus,[26] infection is rare and the American Association of Gynecological Laparoscopists survey for 1982 showed an abdominal wall or peritoneal cavity infection rate of 3 per 1000.[27] None the less adequate skin preparation and sterilization is essential since cases of necrotizing fasciitis following diagnostic laparoscopy have been reported. The risk factors for this potentially fatal infection include old age, obesity and diabetes.[28]

Leakage of ascitic fluid

This is best prevented by careful suture of the wound by full thickness non-absorbable sutures in all patients with massive ascites. When it occurs, the application of a bag in the expectation that the leakage will dry up is both unwarranted and dangerous, since the risk of infection of the peritoneal cavity is high in these patients. Formal closure under aseptic conditions should be performed without delay.

Omental prolapse/Richter's hernia

This results from removing the cannula too rapidly, before the peritoneal cavity has been adequately desufflated. When complete, a tongue of omental tissue is dragged out beyond skin level by the cannula. The prolapsed omental tissue should be carefully replaced by a dissecting forceps. A more serious situation arises when the prolapsed omentum, or much more rarely small bowel, does not reach the skin surface and is therefore not observed. It may then be included in the suture used to close the abdominal stab wound. If a knuckle of bowel is trapped in this way, strangulation and peritonitis will ensue postoperatively.

REFERENCES

1   Ruddock, J.C. (1957) Peritoneoscopy. *Surg. Clin. N. Am. 37:* 1249–1253.
2   Zoeckler, S.J. (1958) Peritoneoscopy. *Gastroenterology, 34:* 969–980.
3   Bruhl, W. (1966) Zwischenfälle und Komplikationen bei der Laparoskopie. *Dt. med. Wschr. 91:* 2297–2299.
4   Wildhirt, E. (1970) Laparoskopie und Leberbiopsie. *Wien. med. Wschr. 120:* 66–69.
5   Villardel, F., Seres, I. & Marti-Vincenti, A. (1967) Complications of peritoneoscopy. A survey of 1455 examinations. *Gastrointest. Endosc. 14:* 178–180.
6   Look, D. (1972) Komplikationen aus 2900 Laparoskopien. *Z. Gastroenterologie. 10:* 437–439.
7   Tadaki, H. & Miura, K. (1974) Peritoneoscopic technics in Japan. In *Gastrointestinal Endoscopy.* Berry, L. (ed.) Chapter 38, pp. 572–586. Springfield, Illinois: Thomas.
8   Berci, G. & Jensen, D. (1982) Laparoscopy for the hepatologist and general surgeon. *Acta Endoscopica, 12:* 3–12.
9   Cuschieri, A. (1980) Laparoscopy in general surgery and gastroenterology. *Br. J. hosp. Med. 24:* 252–258.
10 Booker, W.M. & Johnson, A. (1944) Pneumoperitoneum: physiological effects. *Anesth. Analg. 2:* 23–26.
11 Elwood, B.J., Piltz, G.F. & Potter, B.P. (1940) Electrocardiographic observations on pneumoperitoneum. *Am. Heart J. 19:* 206–208.
12 Gordon, N.L.M., Smith, I. & Shwapp, G.H. (1972) Cardiac arrhythmias during laparoscopy. *Br. med. J. i:* 625.
13 Scott, D.B. & Julian, D.G. (1972) Observations on cardiac arrhythmias during laparoscopy. *Br. med. J. i:* 411–413.
14 Motew, M., Ivancovich, A., Bieniac, J. et al. (1973) Cardiovascular effects and acid–base and blood gases during laparoscopy. *Am. J. Obstet. Gynec. 115:* 1002–1012.
15 Lenz, R.J., Thomas, T.A. & Wilkins, D.G. (1976) Cardiovascular changes during laparoscopy. *Anaesthesia, 31:* 4–12.
16 Carmichael, D.E. (1970) Laparoscopy: cardiac considerations. *Fert. Steril. 22:* 69–70.
17 El-Miawi, M.F., Wahbi, O., El-Bagouri, I.S. et al. (1981) Physiologic changes during CO_2 and N_2O pneumoperitoneum in diagnostic laparoscopy. *J. repro. Med. 26:* 338–346.
18 Hodgson, C., McClelland, N. & Newton, J.R. (1970) Some effects of the peritoneal insufflation of carbon dioxide at laparoscopy. *Anaesthesia, 25:* 382–390.

19 Scott, D.B. (1972) Cardiac arrhythmias during laparoscopy. *Br. med. J. ii:* 49–50.

20 Sharp, J.R., Pierson, W.P. & Brady III, C.E. (1982) Comparison of CO_2- and N_2O-induced discomfort during peritoneoscopy under local anaesthesia. *Gastroenterology. 82:* 453–456.

21 Chamberlain, G. & Brown, J.C. (1982) *Gynaecological Laparoscopy. The Report of a Working Party in a Confidential Enquiry of Gynaecological Laparoscopy.* London: *Royal College of Obstetricians and Gynaecologists.*

22 Graff, T.D., Arbgast, N.R., Phillips, O.C. et al. (1959) Gas embolism. A comparative study of air and carbon dioxide as embolic agents in the systemic venous system. *Am. J. Obstet. Gynec. 78:* 259–265.

23 Wadhwa, R.K., McKenzie, S.R., Wadhwa, D.L. et al. (1978) Gas embolism during laparoscopy. *Anaesthesiology, 48:* 74–76.

24 Yacoub, O.F., Cardona, I., Coveler, L.A. et al. (1982) Carbon dioxide embolism during laparoscopy. *Anaesthesiology, 57:* 533–535.

25 McKenzie, R. (1971) Laparoscopy. *N.Z. Med. J. 74:* 87–91.

26 Carson, S.L., Dole, M., Kraus, R. et al. (1979) Studies in sterilization of the laparoscope: II. *J. repro. Med. 23:* 57.

27 Phillips, S.M., Hulka, J.F. & Petersen, J. (1982) American Association of Gynecologic Laparoscopists 1982 Membership Survey. *J. repro. Med. 29:* 592–594.

28 Sortel, G., Hirsch, E. & Edelin, K. (1983) Necrotizing fasciitis following diagnostic laparoscopy. *Obstet. Gynec. 62:* 67–69 (Suppl.).

29 Zimmerman, H.G. (1982) *Chirurgische Laparoskopie.* Heidelberg: Springer-Verlag.

Index